The Rainforest Mec

CHANCA PIEDRA

(*"Stone-Breaker" Phyllanthus niruri*)

NATURE'S SECRET FOR KIDNEY STONES

LESLIE TAYLOR, ND

Bestselling Author of *The Healing Power of Rainforest Herbs*

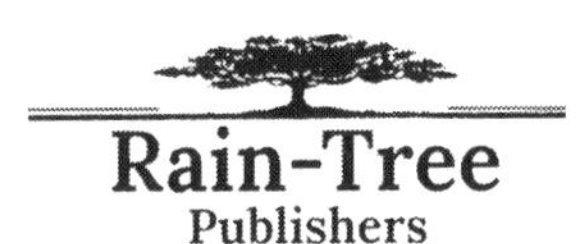

The information and advice contained in this book are based upon the research and the professional experiences of the author, and are not intended as a substitute for consulting with a healthcare professional. The publisher and author are not responsible for any adverse effects or consequences resulting from the use of any of the suggestions discussed in this book. All matters pertaining to your physical health, including your diet and supplement routine, should be supervised by a healthcare professional who can provide medical care that is tailored to meet your individual needs.

Published by

Rain-Tree Publishers

Bullard, Texas 75757

www.rain-tree.com

ISBN: 978-1-7346847-4-2

Cover and Interior Production by Gary A. Rosenberg

www.thebookcouple.com

About the Rainforest Medicinal Plant Guide Series

This book is part of Leslie Taylor's Rainforest Medicinal Plant Guide series featuring the important medicinal plants of the rainforest that she has studied and used for more than 20 years. These guides provide factual, scientific, and vital information on how to use these powerful medicinal plants effectively to improve your health.

The author sells no herbal supplements or products other than books. The books in this series do not promote any specific brands or herbal supplement products. These definitive plant guides concern the plants and their researched effective actions and uses. The information in these guides is more extensive, complete, and unbiased than natural product companies who sell these plants as supplements can provide.

More information on Leslie Taylor's background, knowledge, and experience can be found on the Rain-Tree website (www.rain-tree.com/author.htm) See the Rain-Tree Publishers book page (www.rain-tree.com/books.htm) to learn when new plant guides in the series are released.

Contents

Introduction

Chanca piedra (*Phyllanthus niruri*) is a powerful medicinal herb from the Amazon rainforest. It has been used to treat kidney stones for generations in the Amazon and in traditional herbal medicine systems in South America. Clinical studies now validate this rainforest plant's ability to treat as well as prevent the reoccurrence of several types of kidney stones. In fact, the name *chanca piedra* is Spanish and translates to "stone breaker" based on this long-standing effective use. If you've ever had a kidney stone, you need to know about chanca piedra!

This book will teach you how to use chanca piedra safely and effectively for kidney stones and gout and, just as important, the strategy and dosages required to prevent them in the future. As a naturopathic practitioner, I have used this remarkable rainforest herbal remedy as my "go-to herb" for kidney stones, gallstones, and gout for more than 20 years. I was overjoyed to see (and share in this book) all the new research conducted on the plant, scientifically explaining the many ways chanca piedra works to expel and prevent stones and treat and prevent gout. In the past, it was hard to explain to my clients how a single herb could reduce the pain of a kidney stone, gallstone, or gout attack with the first couple of capsules or cup of herbal tea so immediately and effectively, and this new research finally explains why.

Like most rainforest medicinal plants, chanca piedra is a storehouse of highly active natural chemical compounds that provide many health benefits. Chanca piedra's ability to treat kidney stones only scratches the surface of its many effective uses. Over the last 10 years, scientists have confirmed that this small but powerful herb is quite effective for treating viral and bacterial infections, malaria and other tropical parasitic diseases, and diabetes, and provides strong liver-protective, heart-protective, immune-modulating, and anti-inflammatory benefits. Some of these benefits are a result of more than 70 natural plant compounds called polyphenols, which have strong antioxidant and anti-inflammatory actions—a number of which are found only in chanca piedra.

Some of the research on chanca piedra revealed in this book is quite timely—the ability of chanca piedra to treat viral infections. As I am writing this book, the world has been turned upside down by a new pandemic virus, COVID-19. After I reviewed all the new research on chanca piedra in preparation of writing this book, it had me reaching for the phone to order chanca piedra for my family and myself just in case we were faced with fighting this new virus.

I've used chanca piedra for many years as an effective herbal antiviral, so that wasn't a surprise. It's been the subject of clinical research in humans over many years to treat hepatitis B and C. It's also been confirmed to be effective against several herpes viruses, HIV, influenza and flu viruses, dengue virus, and others. The accumulation of a great deal of research over the years confirms that chanca piedra can kill viruses in people, animals, and plants.

Scientist have reported several different mechanisms of actions for how this powerful little herb kills viruses. One significant mechanism is by inhibiting enzymes and other substances viruses need to divide and multiply (transcriptase and protease), while also providing a direct toxic effect to some viruses (as well as bacteria). Researchers have confirmed the presence of at least eight natural plant chemicals with antiviral actions in the plant. It has not been scientifically tested against this particular coronavirus yet, but it certainly has potential since it's been shown to kill other flu viruses. But that's not the only reason I ordered chanca piedra for my family and myself.

In addition to being a good antiviral, significant new research on chanca piedra confirms it is an effective immune modulator. This is highly important information in regard to this particular coronavirus. Unlike other flu viruses, COVID-19 causes a radical immune system reaction that sends pro-inflammatory chemicals (called cytokines) to the lungs, resulting in severe lung inflammation, which can cause immediate lung tissue damage and cell death. This phenomenon has been termed a "cytokine storm," and when this storm occurs in some people with the virus, hospitalization for breathing assistance becomes necessary. Research shows that chanca piedra has the potential ability to prevent or interrupt this cytokine storm with proven immunomodulatory actions, which I find quite compelling.

Remarkably, research on chanca piedra reveals that it can significantly increase the production and activation of specific immune cells responsible for killing foreign invaders (like viruses and bacteria), while lowering the production of immune cells and cytokines that cause inflammation—the very same cytokines implicated in a COVID-19 cytokine storm. This ability has been confirmed in human research. In patients with pneumonia, asthma, and tuberculosis who were studied, a significant reduction in lung inflammation was noted with significantly lower levels of pro-inflammatory cytokines, which cause lung inflammation, oxidative stress, cellular damage, and cell death. In addition, adults and children with pneumonia, tuberculosis, hepatitis, chicken pox, and Hanson's disease (leprosy) mounted a much stronger immune response to fight these infections, which sped healing and viral/bacterial clearance, when using chanca piedra. It was also noted in these clinical studies that immune cells responsible for immunity were also increased, and those taking chanca piedra for their infections had no relapses or secondary infections and had higher levels of antigens (cells responsible for immunity).

Chanca piedra's many strong antioxidant plant chemicals were probably one reason for this reduction of lung inflammation and lung damage; however, other research has been published on chanca piedra's effective anti-inflammatory actions delivered by other novel anti-inflammatory chemicals. At this juncture, I don't know if or how chanca piedra might treat this new emerging virus, but the research I read was promising enough that I would certainly try it if I were to become infected. In fact, it would be the first natural remedy I would reach for. I know well the safety of chanca piedra—no toxicity, side effects, or other ill effects have been reported in any of the human and animal studies thus far, so it certainly would be worth a try.

Scientists and doctors around world have been concerned about new emerging infectious diseases for quite a few years now. Bacteria, viruses, fungi, and even the parasites like those that cause malaria have been mutating and creating drug resistance to most of our gold-standard drugs. These "superbugs" may well be a much more common problem in our future, and it is certainly impacting us right now. The rainforests of the world are, and will continue to be, of the most utmost importance and one of the main areas where the search for new antimicrobial drugs is taking place. Rainforests hold the highest biodiversity and sheer number of novel chemicals on the planet. Acre for acre, there are more species of plants, animals, insects, and even microbial species such as bacteria, fungi, and viruses in the rainforests than anywhere else on earth.

In the species-rich rainforest, there are many different types of fungi, mold, bacteria, viruses, and parasites, as well as hordes of insects that attack and kill plants. It is of little wonder that rainforest plants contain so many potent, active, and defensive plant chemicals—they are in a constant battle for survival in an environment literally teeming with life that is constantly evolving. From the soil-borne root-rot (a virus) that attacks tender herbaceous plants, to the fungi and mold smothering the life out of huge canopy trees or even the incredible amount of insects devouring any defenseless leaf in the forest . . . rainforest plants have learned to adapt, create chemical defenses against attack and to survive.

Within this rich arsenal of defensive chemicals, many rainforest plants like chanca piedra have been tested with antibacterial, antiviral, antifungal, antiparasitic, anti-mold, and insecticidal chemicals with potent actions. In fact, you'll learn in this book that chanca piedra has also been reported to kill multidrug-resistant bacteria and drug-resistant malaria in test-tube studies and/or in animal studies. It is likely that within these diverse chemicals created to protect the plants from disease, at least a handful of highly active chemicals can and will be harvested and put to the use of protecting humans and animals from the same types of disease-causing organisms. Chanca piedra has been targeted within this search for active chemicals capable of killing microorganisms, and research is ongoing on several active natural compounds in chanca piedra.

This is important information to know! My goal in writing this book is to share the information on what the new research reveals about chanca piedra and how to use it effectively and safely for kidney stones, viral and bacterial infections, liver and gallbladder problems, and other conditions. I'll share my naturopathic protocols I've used for more than 20 years on effective dosages in the upcoming chapters, as well as other important information on how to choose a good product and how to use chanca piedra as an effective rainforest herbal remedy. Chanca piedra has long been in my personal arsenal of effective herbal remedies and will continue to be long into the future. I am excited to share with you everything I've learned recently and over many years using this powerful and especially important rainforest remedy.

CHAPTER 1

What Is Chanca Piedra?

Chanca piedra is a small, erect, annual herb that is indigenous to the rainforests of the Amazon and other tropical areas throughout the world, including South America, Africa, India, and China. Chanca piedra is quite prevalent in the Amazon and other wet rainforests, growing and spreading freely, much like a weed.

Its botanical name is *Phyllanthus niruri.* Unfortunately, there has been a great deal of confusion among scientists regarding the plant's botanical name, and, in many cases, plant misidentification makes evaluation of published information difficult. *Phyllanthus amarus* and *Phyllanthus sellowianus* are often considered varieties of *Phyllanthus niruri,* or no distinction is made among these three species in published clinical research. Oftentimes, one name is indicated to be synonymous with another, and, sometimes, both names are used interchangeably as if referring to one plant. It became so confusing that, in the 1990s, a major reorganization of the *Phyllanthus* genus was conducted, which classified *Phyllanthus amarus* as a variety of *Phyllanthus niruri.* The new accepted botanical name for *Phyllanthus amarus* is *Phyllanthus niruri var. amarus. Phyllanthus amarus* and *Phyllanthus sellowianus* are closely related to *Phyllanthus niruri* in appearance, phytochemical structure, and history of use, but typically are found in the drier tropical climates of India, Brazil, and even Florida and Texas.

Chanca piedra is the name of the plant in Peru and other Spanish-speaking countries in South America. The English translation of the name is "stone breaker," and it refers to the plant's very long history of use in the treatment of kidney stones. In Brazil, the Portuguese name is *quebra pedra,* which translates to "break stone," or *arranca-pedras,* which means "shatter stone." Wherever the plant is grown, it usually has a local common name by which it is referred to. Since chanca piedra was originally introduced into the American natural products market as chanca piedra, most available products or supplements sold in the United States today use "chanca piedra" or "stone breaker" on their labels.

The *Phyllanthus* genus contains more than 1,000 species of shrubs, trees, and annual or biennial herbs distributed throughout the tropical and subtropical regions of both hemispheres. Many *Phyllanthus* plants are used as traditional medicines; chanca piedra is the most well known.

Chanca piedra is a weedy annual herb that grows about one to two feet high. It bears numerous ascending herbaceous green branches, or stems. Small bright lime-green leaves grow on each side of the stem in an alternating pattern. Pale green flowers, often tinged with red, are produced on the underside of the stem. The flowers become tiny fruits—smooth capsules containing seeds, which grow under the leaves. For this reason, one of chanca piedra's common names is "seed-under-leaf."

Traditional Uses in Herbal Medicine

Chanca piedra was named for its effective use by generations of Amazonian indigenous people for eliminating gallstones and kidney stones. In addition to kidney stones, the plant is employed in the Amazon for numerous other conditions by the indigenous people, including colic, diabetes, malaria, dysentery, fever, flu, tumors, jaundice, vaginitis, gonorrhea, and dyspepsia. Based on its long-documented history of use in the region, the plant is also generally employed to reduce pain, expel intestinal gas, stimulate and promote digestion, expel worms, and as a mild laxative.

Various species of *Phyllanthus* plants have been used in Ayurvedic medicine in India for over 2,000 years with a wide number of traditional uses. These include employing the whole plant for jaundice, diabetes, gonorrhea, frequent menstruation, leprosy, asthma, bronchitis, fevers, and various urogenital diseases. It is also used topically as a poultice for skin ulcers, sores, swelling, wounds, and itchiness. The *Phyllanthus niruri* species is used as an ingredient in almost 175 different Ayurvedic formulations in India today.

Chanca piedra has a long history in herbal medicine systems in every tropical country where it grows. For the most part, it is used for similar conditions worldwide. In addition to kidney stones, its main uses are for many types of liver and urinary conditions and infections; for gallstones; for hepatitis, colds, flu, tuberculosis, and other viral infections; liver diseases and disorders, including anemia, jaundice, and liver cancer; and for bacterial infections such as cystitis, prostatitis, venereal diseases, and urinary tract infections. It is also widely employed for diabetes and hypertension as well as for its diuretic, pain-relieving, digestive-stimulant, antispasmodic, fever-reducing, and cellular-protective properties in many other conditions.

Current Uses as an Herbal Remedy

Chanca piedra has been sold as a single-herb herbal remedy in the United States and Europe since 1995. It is a well-established and respected natural remedy to break up and expel both kidney stones and gallstones. It is believed to help stimulate the production of bile and to promote healthy liver and gallbladder function as well as to treat disorders in the gallbladder, liver, and kidneys. It is typically used as a stand-alone therapy for kidney stones and to treat liver disorders, while it is usually combined with other herbs for the treatment of gallstones. In the alternative and integrative health practitioners' market, chanca piedra is also used for various viral infections, including hepatitis B and C. In Germany, where common herbal supplements are classified as herbal drugs that require a doctor's prescription, chanca piedra is a patented herbal drug for hepatitis; it's also available in a few other European countries for that purpose.

Natural Compounds and Chemicals

Since the mid-1960s, chanca piedra has been the subject of a great deal of phytochemical research to determine its active constituents and their pharmacological activities. More than 130 natural chemical compounds have been identified in chanca piedra. It is a rich source of plant chemicals, including many that have been found only in the *Phyllanthus* genus. Many of the active constituents are attributed to biologically active compounds found in the leaf, stem, and root of the plant, including lignans, glycosides, flavonoids, alkaloids, phenols, ellagitannins, saponins, steroidal sapogenins, and terpenoids. Common lipids and fatty acids also occur in the plant. Many of chanca piedra's flavonoids, phenols, and ellagitannins have been documented in a great deal of research to be strong antioxidants that can fight free radicals, reduce levels of reactive oxygen species (ROS), and relieve oxidative stress in several different ways. These natural compounds fall into a large category of plant compounds called polyphenols. Polyphenols are discussed in much more detail in the next chapter.

In a recent study, just 1 gram of dried chanca piedra was shown to contain 203 milligrams of polyphenols, 18 milligrams of terpenoids, and 12 milligrams of saponins. These documented levels can vary in published research depending on how researchers extract the plant to test it for these chemicals. The compounds studied in chanca piedra are documented with various pharmacological actions: lignans have excellent liver-protective and antiviral properties, whereas terpenes exhibited anticancer and antimicrobial activity. Flavonoids showed strong antioxidant activity, and the alkaloids exhibited antispasmodic, antimicrobial, and pain-relieving activity.

While many find the subject of chemistry tedious, the chemistry of a plant directly relates to the main actions and benefits the plant provides as an herbal remedy. Chanca piedra certainly has some interesting chemistry since it contains some chemicals that are found only in this plant or in closely related *Phyllanthus* plants species.

Ethnic Medicinal Uses of Chanca Piedra	
Amazonia	For bowel inflammation, colic, constipation, diabetes, digestion stimulation, dysentery, dyspepsia, edema, fever, flu, gallstones, gonorrhea, intestinal gas, itch, jaundice, kidney aliments, kidney stones, malaria, pain, proctitis, stomachaches, tumor, urinary insufficiency, urinary tract disorders, vaginitis, and worms; to stimulate menstruation
Bahamas/ Caribbean	For bacterial infections, colds, constipation, fever, flu, hypoglycemic, laxative, liver detoxifier, liver tonic, liver protector, spasms, stomachache, typhoid, urinary insufficiency, and viral infections; as an appetite stimulant
Brazil	For abortions, aches (joint), albuminuria, arthritis, bacterial infections, bile stimulant, biliary conditions, bladder problems, bladder stones, blood cleanser, cancer, colds and flu, catarrh (liver and kidney), cystitis, diabetes, digestion stimulation, edema, fever, gallbladder stimulation, gallstones, gastritis, gastrointestinal problems, gout, hepatitis, hypertension, hypoglycemic, inflammation, jaundice, kidney colic, kidney pain, kidney stones, liver support, liver disorders, malaria, obesity, pain, prostatitis, renal colic, renal problems, spasms, tonic, uric acid excess, urinary insufficiency, urinary problems, uterine relaxant, and viral infections; as a muscle relaxant and to promote perspiration
Haiti	For bowel inflammation, colic, digestive problems, digestion stimulation, fever, flu, indigestion, intestinal gas, malaria, spasms, stomachache, and urinary insufficiency
India	For anemia, asthma, bronchitis, colds and flu, conjunctivitis, cough, diabetes, diarrhea, digestion stimulation, dysentery, fevers, edema, eye disorders, flu, genitourinary disorders, gonorrhea, hepatitis, jaundice, kidney stones, lack of milk production, menstrual disorders, ringworm, scabies, thirst, tuberculosis, tumor (abdomen), urinary insufficiency, urogenital tract infections, vaginal discharge, and warts
Malaysia	For caterpillar stings, constipation, dermatosis, diarrhea, itch, kidney stones, menstruation promoter, miscarriage, renal disorders, syphilis, urinary insufficiency, and vertigo

Peru	For gallstones, gout, hepatitis, kidney pain, kidney problems, kidney stones, liver disorders, urinary infections, viral infections, and worms; to stimulate menstruation
United States	For bile insufficiency, bronchitis, colds and flu, diabetes, fever, gallbladder problems, gallstones, gout, hepatitis, hypertension, kidney problems, kidney stones, liver disease, obstructions, pain, uric acid excess, urinary tract infections, and viral infections
Elsewhere	For bile insufficiency, bruises, colds and flu, constipation, cough, cuts, diabetes, diarrhea, dysentery, dyspepsia, edema, eye diseases, fever, gallstones, gonorrhea, itch, jaundice, kidney disease, kidney stones, malaria, menstrual problems, pain, rectitis, stomachache, tuberculosis, urinary insufficiency, urinary tract infections, vaginitis, venereal diseases, and viruses

The plant chemistry of chanca piedra is a perfect example of nature's synergy in a medicinal plant. While many of the individual plant compounds and natural chemicals are the subject of research to determine their individual actions and benefits, researchers have noted repeatedly that there is a synergy, or additive effect, of these chemicals working together. The actions and benefits of chanca piedra, which contains all the chemicals working together synergistically, is reported in many studies to be much greater than the action of any isolated single chemical. For example, several novel chemicals in chanca piedra have shown anti-inflammatory actions, but the whole plant has more than 20 natural anti-inflammatory compounds that work together synergistically to relieve inflammation. When chanca piedra was tested in animals and in test tubes, the anti-inflammatory action of the natural leaf or whole plant was stronger than any single plant compound tested.

In much of the research conducted on chanca piedra, researchers attributed the beneficial actions they were observing to several chemicals, which was certainly true for the plant's antiviral actions against hepatitis. Most plant research in the United States is funded by drug companies looking for novel plant chemicals with beneficial actions that they can turn into profitable new drugs. Once they target a chemical or two in a plant they're studying, all the focus and research shifts to the targeted chemicals rather than the whole plant they found the chemical in. However, in the case of chanca piedra's antiviral actions, the results of the whole herb natural remedy (with its many chemicals working together) kept fueling research on the plant as a whole instead of on any single antiviral plant chemical it contains.

Research has determined that the main active plant chemicals in chanca piedra include the following: 1-O-galloyl-6-O-luteoyl-α-D-glucose, 4-methoxy-nor-securinine, 5-demethoxy-niranthin, allo-securine, amariinic acid, amariin, amarosterol A & B, amarulone, astragalin, beta-sitosterol, brevifolin, brevifolin carboxylic acid, chlorogenic acid, corilagin, cymene, dihydrosecurinine, demethylenedioxy-niranthin, diosgenin, elaeocarpusin, ellagic acid, epibubbialine, eridictyol-7-rhamnopyranoside, fisetin-4-O-glucoside, farnesyl-farnesol derivatives, friedelin, furosin, gallic acid, gallocatechin, geraniin, geraniinic acid B, glucogallin, hinokinin, heliobupthalmin lactones, hydroxyniranthin, hypophyllanthin, isobubbialine, isocorilagin, isoquercitrin, isolintetralin, isonirtetralin, kaempferol, kaempferol 3-O-d-glucopyranoside, linalool, linnanthin, linolenic acid, lintetralin, lupeol, methyl salicylate, norsecurinine, niranthin, nirphyllin, nirtetralin, niruretin, nirurin, nirurine, niruriside, norsecurinines, oleanolic acid, orthosiphol I and G, phenazine, phyllamyricin D-F, phyllamyricoside A-C, phyllantheol, phyllanthin, phyllanthine, phyllanthenol, phyllanthenone, phyllanthusiin A-D, phyllochrysine, phytetralin, phyltetralin, quercetin, quercetin-3-O-glucopyranoside, quercetin, quercetol, quercitrin, repandusinic acid A & B, ricinoleic acid, rutin, saponins, securinol, securinine, tetrahydrosecurinine, triacontanal, tricontanol, urinatetralin, ursolic acid, and virgatusin.

CHAPTER 2

The Power of Polyphenols

Polyphenols are a large classification of naturally occurring plant compounds found in all medicinal plants as well as in fruits and vegetables. Some polyphenolic compounds are quite common and can be found in varying degrees in almost all plants. Chanca piedra is unusual because it produces a number of novel polyphenols that are found only in this plant and others that occur only in closely related species of *Phyllanthus* medicinal plants. Unlike other common plants, chanca piedra also delivers a significant amount of polyphenol compounds, which can result in therapeutic levels with medicinal actions. You'll learn in this chapter why polyphenols are important and how they contribute to the documented actions and benefits of chanca piedra.

What Is a Polyphenol?

We've known about plant polyphenols for quite a few years, and they've been studied extensively. Over 80,000 research studies have been published on polyphenols since the mid-1980s, and research continues today at a fast pace. More than 8,000 different polyphenols have been identified thus far, and we continue to discover new ones, mostly in medicinal plants and novel tropical fruits.

Polyphenols are unique natural plant compounds that can be found in all plants and, typically, almost all parts of the plants—leaves, stems, barks, fruits, fruit peels or skin, seeds, and roots. Every plant contains a unique combination of polyphenols, which is why different plants and fruits, all rich in these substances, can have very different effects on the body.

All living things have inbred survival instincts. It is literally part of the cellular makeup of all species on earth. In highly mobile species like humans and other animals, the main survival instinct and mechanism is "flee, fight, or hide." Even bacteria and virus species have learned to flee or hide from immune cells and chemical agents attacking them, as well as to fight them by mutating or changing their own physical structure to defend against them. With stationary plants rooted to the ground and incapable of physically fleeing from danger, their survival instinct is controlled by wonderfully complex and rich chemical defense mechanisms that have evolved over eons. Plants have either created a chemical defense mechanism against what might harm them, or they have succumbed and become extinct. This is the mechanism the plants use to survive, grow, and flourish as well as to fight the many disease-causing organisms that attack them. Creating and utilizing polyphenols is one of the main mechanisms plants use to survive, grow, and flourish, to fight the many disease-causing organisms that attack them, as well as repair the damage they've caused.

Polyphenols are created in plants as a part of a plant's unique biochemical immune system and antioxidant system. These chemicals reduce free radicals and prevent or repair the damage caused by free radicals that the plants are exposed to. Oxidative damage in plants can be a result of less than perfect growing conditions, soil toxins and heavy metals, too much or too little water, too much or too little sunlight, and other negative conditions. Polyphenols are also the healing and repairing agents in plants' specialized "immune systems" to overcome and heal damage by insects and browsing animals, and to protect it from various microbes like plant viruses, bacteria, fungi, and mold.

This is why the type and number of polyphenols can vary widely in plants and the same plants can vary in polyphenol levels from one growing season to another. It really all depends on what types of damage and negative growing conditions the plants had to overcome by increasing its polyphenol content. The more stressful conditions, the higher the polyphenol content. It is also for this reason that wild-harvested plants usually have more polyphenols than cultivated plants. Growers of cultivated plants, like fruits and vegetables and even medicinal plants, control stress factors to their crops to increase harvesting yields . . . from proper irrigation, added soil nutrients, insect control, and even protection from intense sunlight. Controlling these factors will result in the plant needing to produce less stress-reducing and healing polyphenols.

These aspects also explain why medicinal plants usually have higher amounts and more diversity in their polyphenol content than either wild-harvested or cultivated medicinal plants in the United States or Europe. The growing conditions in the tropics are just more intense and stressful. High humidity (which promotes more mold and fungi), intense heat and sunlight, and periods of monsoon-like rains followed by dry periods in the typical rainy-dry seasons of the tropics all contribute to the need of tropical plants to increase polyphenol production to protect themselves. And let's not forget about the bugs! Without a cold season to kill off crawling bugs as well as bacteria, viruses, and fungi, the diversity of pests that tropical plants are exposed to are much higher in the tropics than in temperate climates. When botanists say a particular plant has "adapted" to grow in the tropics, this adaptation is usually all about the plant's having increased its natural polyphenol production enough to survive in these more extreme growing conditions.

Another interesting aspect regarding polyphenols and plants as it relates to chanca piedra is that chanca piedra is classified as a weed. Just like most weeds, it is hard to kill because its survival mechanisms, and resulting polyphenols, are numerous and strong. Chanca piedra joins the ranks of other medicinal plants like dandelion, nettles, dock, elecampane, mullein, and many other common North American plants that are classified as weeds. They are all hard to eradicate because of the healing, repairing, and protective polyphenols they manufacture. As most gardeners are quick to note, when poor growing conditions negatively affect their beloved flowers and vegetables, the weeds adapt and flourish!

How Polyphenols Are Unique

The main feature that makes a polyphenol a polyphenol is its unique molecular structure, which usually makes them easy to identify. The manner in which the compound is put together molecularly facilitates a polyphenol to easily attach to and bond to other molecules and chemicals, oftentimes creating brand-new compounds. This unique molecular structure also makes polyphenols especially attracted to enzyme chemicals. However, rather than creating a new compound, they often bond to the enzyme and then disable the enzyme from performing its job, making them effective enzyme inhibitors.

For example, one of the reasons most polyphenols have antioxidant actions is that polyphenols are capable of binding with and interfering with two enzymes that are required in the complicated biochemical chain of events that creates a free radical, and especially ROS free radicals. Another good example is this: Some polyphenols are reported with weight loss or blood sugar–lowering actions because those polyphenols bond to and disable the digestive enzymes we produce during digestion that break down sugars and starches in our meals. If these enzymes don't do their job, then the sugar and starches (and their calories) are not broken down and absorbed (raising blood sugar levels and promoting weight gain), and they are eliminated undigested. Not all polyphenols can provide this benefit/action, but some can.

Polyphenols can bind with almost any type of compound—with sugars, with other plant chemicals, and even with each other. These types of new compounds are usually called derivatives or isomers of the chemical a polyphenol connected with. For example, there are two very common natural acids found in many fruits, vegetables, and medicinal plants called caffeic acid and quinic acid. When these two chemicals bind with one another, they create new chemicals that are basically combinations or bonds between these two plant chemicals. These bonds form isomers. One very well-known isomer of caffeic and quinic acids is chlorogenic acid (CGA). So far, more than 71 different CGA compounds have been reported and are widely distributed in plants. These various compounds are just slightly different derivatives of caffeic acid bonding with quinic acid, but actions, benefits, and absorption of these derivatives can be very different.

The binding action of polyphenols can happen inside plants to make more healing and antioxidant chemicals when the plant needs them, and these bonds can happen and new chemicals are formed inside our bodies during digestion. These types of chemicals are called metabolites—a product of metabolism. Unbelievably, while scientists have confirmed there are more than 8,000 unique polyphenols, they estimate that between 100,000 and 200,000 metabolites of polyphenols are created in plants, animals, humans, and even microbes like bacteria.

This makes it harder for scientists to study since digestive processes are so unique, very difficult to create inside a test tube, are often different in laboratory animals than in humans, and are even different among individual humans. To make matters more complicated, some of these polyphenols are not easily digested, and they make it to the colon where we each have our own unique ratio of thousands of gut bacteria species that make up our gut microbiome. Landmark research over the last five years has shown that polyphenols interacting with bacteria in the gut microbiome make a whole host of new chemicals that contribute to many physiological functions. From chemicals that control our appetite, insulin sensitivity, fat storage, fat burning, and inflammation levels to the manufacture of neurotransmitters we need for mood, brain function, and much more, polyphenols are now thought to be the best way to modulate our gut bacteria to promote health.

We will probably never know the total effect polyphenols and their many isomers, derivatives, and metabolites have on promoting heath and treating diseases, but scientists agree, it's a fascinating subject that promotes rigorous ongoing research on these important natural compounds.

Polyphenol Profiles Results in Different Actions

Every plant has its own unique blend of polyphenols. The number of different polyphenols and how much of each of these polyphenols occur make up a plant's unique polyphenol profile. Another important aspect in a plant's polyphenol profile is the synergistic actions polyphenols are known for. For example, while chanca piedra may have only a very small amount of a single well-known antiviral polyphenol, it is working synergistically with a dozen other polyphenols with antiviral actions, as well as other antiviral alkaloid chemicals, which produces a much stronger overall antiviral action than a small amount of just one particular chemical. This also negates the need to use large quantities of a single chemical, which usually results in more side effects. As herbalists and natural health practitioners know, the synergy among many chemicals in lower dosages can provide an equal or greater effect than a single-chemical drug, usually without the side effects of a single chemical in high dosages. With the growing knowledge of the medical benefits of polyphenols, plant researchers and drug researchers are learning to first evaluate a medicinal plant's polyphenol profile for initial clues as to what a plant might treat, prevent, or have a beneficial effect on. A polyphenol profile of a medicinal plant often confirms many of the traditional uses the plant is known for as an herbal remedy.

How Polyphenols Fight Free Radicals

Many people understand that antioxidants "fights free radicals," but most don't realize that antioxidants can work in four different ways. Substances called free radicals, and particularly a group of free radicals called reactive oxygen species (ROS), are a product of normal life, created by metabolizing foods and even the oxygen we breathe into cellular energy, as well as various other chemical interactions in our bodies, which are quite normal. Free radicals are formed when the molecules involved in these processes lose an electron. They travel around the body in search of a new electron to make a pair, thereby causing damage.

Our bodies have a natural built-in system that is supposed to keep ROS in check and at healthy levels. This includes natural chemicals we produce in our bodies called antioxidants, and they are capable of scavenging or deactivating ROS. Most of the antioxidants we produce, as well as the vitamin antioxidants we consume (vitamins A, C, and E) effectively disable these free radicals by lending them one of their own electrons. This converts the free radical into a stable molecule again.

Unfortunately, many diseases, health conditions, and internal deregulations can occur that greatly increases ROS, which can then overwhelm or disable our natural antioxidant system. Other things can limit our ability to produce these antioxidants. For example, just eating too much sugar (especially high-fructose corn syrup, which is found in soda) reduces our bodies' ability to produce our own natural antioxidant chemicals to keep ROS at healthy levels. If we produce too much ROS or our natural antioxidant system becomes overwhelmed or fails, the result is oxidative stress.

Oxidative stress can damage many different types of cells and organs. ROS and free radicals are particularly damaging to the cells in the heart and cardiovascular system because they are actually circulating in our bloodstream. Thousands of studies report the mechanisms by which ROS can contribute to the development of clogged arteries, high blood pressure, peripheral vascular disease, coronary artery disease, cardiomyopathy, heart failure, and cardiac arrhythmias.

When cells suffer oxidative stress, inflammation results and, left untreated, even more cellular damage occurs. When oxidative stress begins to damage cells, the immune system gets triggered to repair or remove the damaged cells, and this results in even more inflammation as well as the generation of even more ROS, which creates a vicious circle. Inflammation is a natural process our immune system uses to repair or eliminate unhealthy cells. Therefore, oxidative stress usually goes hand in hand with inflammation, and it can result in a chronic low-level state of inflammation throughout our bodies. This can negatively impact various organs and internal processes. If you have never heard of ROS, free radicals, and/or antioxidants, you might find another book in the Rainforest Plant Guide Series helpful: *Acerola: Nature's Secret to Fight Free Radicals.*

It explains how natural plant antioxidants react with free radicals, including ROS, to relieve oxidative stress and chronic inflammation in much greater detail. Visit Amazon.com or the Rain-Tree website for more information on how to obtain the book.

Almost without exception, polyphenols are widely documented as strong antioxidants. Not only can they quench free radicals, but they have cellular-protective effects to protect cells and organs from the damaging oxidation and resulting cellular damage that free radicals cause. Utilizing their binding actions with enzymes, polyphenols interfere in the chemical chain of events that's required to make a free radical. Some polyphenols can also encourage the production of our own natural antioxidant enzymes to help address free radicals.

The powerful antioxidant nature of polyphenols has been demonstrated repeatedly in research to prevent or treat various diseases and conditions where oxidative stress is a factor in the development or progression of the disease—of which there are many. In addition, polyphenols are typically called "chain-breaking" antioxidants and are very important to add to vitamin antioxidants like vitamin C. When vitamin C lends an electron to a free radical, it becomes a pro-oxidant itself, and with two missing electrons, it can actually become a free radical, causing cellular damage until it is quenched by another antioxidant. When polyphenols lend electrons, they remain fairly stable and so prevent the initiation of further radical reactions. Polyphenols can also lend electrons to unstable vitamin C intermediates and "break the chain" reaction of vitamins turning from antioxidants to pro-oxidants to free radicals.

The Main Actions of Polyphenols

While every natural plant chemical has unique actions and benefits, polyphenol compounds generally share some common properties and actions (in addition to providing highly effective antioxidant actions). These are detailed next. As you'll learn, many of these actions are actually the result of the reduction of oxidative stress and the chronic inflammation it causes.

Anti-inflammatory Actions

When most people think of inflammation, they think of the body's temporary response to injury and infection—a response that can be painful, but is an essential part of the body's healing process. Unfortunately, not all inflammation is beneficial to the body. To understand why, we have to look at the difference between acute and chronic inflammation and how free radicals cause chronic inflammation.

Acute inflammation is where our immune system shines. When we suffer an injury, such as a sprained ankle, chemical messengers known as cytokines are released by the damaged tissue and cells at the site of injury. These cytokines act as "emergency signals" that send out more of the body's immune cells, hormones, and nutrients. Blood vessels dilate and blood flow increases so that the healing agents can move quickly into the blood to flood the injured area. This inflammatory response is what causes the ankle to turn red and become swollen. As the healing agents go to work, the ankle is repaired, and the inflammation gradually subsides.

Long-term, or chronic, inflammation is different from

acute inflammation, and it's where our immune system and our natural inflammatory processes can cause problems. Chronic inflammation is also called persistent, low-grade inflammation because it can produce a steady, low level of inflammation throughout the body. This condition has been proven to contribute to many diseases, and research suggests it may cause some common chronic diseases such as diabetes, heart diseases, and even aging. Low levels of inflammation can be triggered by a perceived internal threat—just as an injury triggers acute inflammation—even when there isn't a disease to fight or an injury to heal. This can activate the body's natural immune response, and inflammation is the result.

The cellular damage caused by free radicals is the main perceived threat in our bodies that activates the immune system to cause inflammation. When healthy cells become damaged or begin dying from free radical damage, the body triggers the immune system to start the inflammatory process in an effort to repair or remove the cells. Because free radicals are distributed throughout the body, and the cellular damage is occurring cell by cell wherever a free radical interacts with a healthy cell, the inflammatory response spreads throughout the body. The cell-by-cell damage is smaller than damage caused by injury or infection, so the inflammation response is much smaller. This results in low levels of chronic inflammation throughout the body as the immune system tries to do its job of cleaning up or repairing free radical–damaged cells.

Unfortunately, when an imbalance occurs between the production of free radicals and the ability of the body to counteract these substances' negative effects, a negative feedback loop can be generated. In some cells and systems in the body, oxidative stress causes inflammation, and the inflammation can trigger the generation of even more free radicals. Then these additional free radicals create more oxidative stress, which causes more inflammation—a vicious cycle is created, and everything become chronic. It is important to understand that this process may have a detrimental effect on every one of our cells and in many of our complicated internal biochemical processes in different organs. This negative cycle can continue silently, usually without any outward symptoms or signs, causing us significant risks of developing chronic disease without even knowing.

While free radical damage can be the biggest cause of chronic inflammation, it's certainly not the only cause. But that's where polyphenol antioxidants can play a huge role and a greater one than vitamin antioxidants and our own natural enzyme antioxidants can. Most all polyphenols have antioxidant and anti-inflammatory actions. Polyphenols work in several ways to reduce and relieve inflammation, not just through reducing free radicals. Whether a problem is created by oxidative stress or chronic inflammation, polyphenols can be effective—if you pick the plants that have the right polyphenol combinations and profiles.

Disease Prevention

Tens of thousands of research studies have been published on chronic inflammation and oxidative stress and the roles they play in numerous diseases. We now know that inflammation and oxidative stress can be a cause or a contributing factor to a wide range of diseases, including almost every chronic disease. From heart diseases, diabetes, Alzheimer's disease, and cancer to high cholesterol levels, autoimmune diseases, and even obesity—chronic inflammation and oxidative stress are playing significant roles. Many of these studies reveal that when you reduce oxidative stress and chronic inflammation, it has a beneficial impact on these conditions. Better yet, if you manage your levels of oxidative stress and chronic inflammation with polyphenol antioxidants, you can avoid developing these many conditions. Polyphenol compounds with antioxidant and anti-inflammatory actions have surfaced in all this research as the most important natural plant compounds available to us that have the ability to help prevent these diseases.

Anti-Aging Actions

A significant number of polyphenols have shown the ability to prolong the life span of laboratory animals in new anti-aging research. Again, free radicals are implicated in the overall aging process in both humans and animals. They can accumulate over the years in our bodies, resulting in state of chronic oxidative stress at old age. This affects not only our skin but also many internal cells, organs, and biochemical processes.

Inside most of our cells are organelles called mitochondria, and they play an integral role in biochemical processes going on inside our cells. Mitochondria, which are often called the powerhouses of cells, act like miniature factories, converting the food we eat into usable energy in the form of a chemical called adenosine triphosphate (ATP). ATP provides energy to fuel a myriad of cellular processes. If there is a biochemical process going on inside a cell, it is typically going on in the mitochondria.

Mitochondria are actually a significant generator of free radicals because free radicals are a byproduct of creating ATP. Each of our cells contains a little bit of vitamin C and antioxidant enzymes, and their role is to help deactivate these mitochondrial-produced free radicals. However, mitochondria can also be a target of free radical damage if our natural antioxidant system isn't doing its job effectively, leading to mitochondrial dysfunction. Research now reports that mitochondrial dysfunction is one of the root causes of aging, and it helps create a state of chronic oxidative stress in the elderly. As our cells age, mitochondria lose their ability to provide cellular energy efficiently and release more free radicals, including ROS, that harm cells.

Significant research on polyphenols has reported that these naturally strong and cellular-protective antioxidant compounds can treat and relieve mitochondrial dysfunction. Restoring mitochondrial function basically renews the cell and allows it to function like it did when it was much younger. This is one method by which polyphenols can deliver an anti-aging effect and why they can prolong life in animal studies. However, another significant factor in aging is the accumulation and damage of other free-radical–like substances called advanced glycation end products (AGEs). AGEs also accumulate in our bodies, cells, and organs as we age, and are considered to be the hallmark of cellular aging. The levels of AGEs in our bodies are now thought to directly relate to how well or poorly we age, as well as which age-related chronic diseases we are at risk for.

Again, the research on these powerful polyphenols are revealing that maybe the best natural compounds on the planet that are capable of reducing AGEs and protecting cells and biochemical processes from their damaging effects are polyphenols. Thousands of studies on polyphenols (including those found in chanca piedra) report the anti-aging benefits these effective compounds can provide. See chapter 5 for more information on AGEs and problems they cause and why chanca piedra was reported in research to provide these anti-AGE and anti-aging benefits.

Diabetes and Metabolic Diseases

Polyphenols from different plant-based sources, including those found in chanca piedra, have been shown to influence glucose metabolism in several ways. These include as inhibition of starch digestion and sugar absorption in the intestine, stimulation of insulin secretion from the pancreatic β-cells, modulation of glucose release from the liver, activation of insulin receptors and glucose uptake in the insulin-sensitive tissues, and modulation of liver glucose output. Many polyphenol-rich plants and foods are promoted as antidiabetic or beneficial for the treatment or prevention type-2 diabetes for these reasons.

Type 2 diabetes is also categorized as a chronic inflammatory disease that is associated with oxidative stress and insulin resistance. The increased production of reactive oxygen species (ROS) or a reduced capacity of the ROS-scavenging antioxidants can lead to abnormal changes in intracellular signaling and result in chronic inflammation and insulin resistance. Prevention of ROS-induced oxidative stress and inflammation can be an important therapeutic strategy to prevent the onset of type 2 diabetes and well as diabetic complications and co-occurring diseases.

New research also reveals that fat cell–produced

adipokines play important roles in glucose metabolism and insulin resistance. It is established through human research that adipokines are deregulated in people with diabetes, and these deregulations are one of the underlying reasons obesity or just being overweight increases the risk of developing type 2 diabetes. Since many of these adipokine deregulations can be remediated with substances that reduce inflammation and oxidative stress, polyphenols have evolved as natural substances that can treat or prevent diabetes.

The initiation and progression of diabetes can also be linked to higher AGE levels in the body and the cellular damage, generation of additional free radicals, and inflammation these AGEs cause.

A significant body of research represents important advances related to influence of polyphenols and polyphenol-rich diets on preventing and managing type 2 diabetes. This research reveals that the main methods of actions polyphenols utilize to prevent diabetes include protection of pancreatic beta cells against glucose toxicity; anti-inflammatory and antioxidant effects; inhibition of digestive enzymes, which decrease starch conversion and sugar absorption; and inhibition of AGE production. Anthocyanin-type polyphenols have also been reported to exhibit antidiabetic properties by reducing blood sugar and HbA1c levels as well as improve insulin secretion and resistance in human and animal studies.

Obesity

New research indicates that obesity is actually a chronic inflammatory disease, and the fatty tissues of overweight individuals are inflamed and suffering from oxidative stress and immune cell damage. When fat cells and fatty tissues are damaged by inflammation and oxidative stress, they do not produce enough of certain natural metabolic chemicals that are required to reduce inflammation, store and burn fats, maintain insulin sensitivity, and support a healthy weight.

Scientists have now discovered more than 80 adipokines that are secreted by fat cells, many of which have known metabolic actions. Research has increased significantly on these natural fat-produced substances and their roles in obesity, diabetes, heart diseases, and other disorders since 2010. New knowledge about these substances and their roles have encouraged the development of new drugs targeting this metabolic system in the treatment of obesity, metabolic diseases, and heart conditions.

Since our fatty tissues and fat cells expand as we gain weight, all these fat-secreted deregulations and resulting inflammation and oxidative stress increases as our fat increases. You don't have to be obese either; just gaining some extra weight can start the process and head you down the road to deregulations. These deregulations make it much harder to lose weight, and some can make it virtually impossible to lose weight. Adipokines also help regulate functions in the heart and how we process sugar and insulin. Obesity-caused adipokine deregulations are now the main link of why obesity significantly increases our risks of developing type 2 diabetes and cardiovascular disease.

We once believed that many of us gained weight as we aged mostly because of reduced activity levels. New research is reporting that the accumulation of free radicals and advanced glycation end products (AGEs) as we age may be the cause of deregulations that promotes weight gain and makes it harder to maintain a healthy weight. Plants that contain strong antioxidant compounds have been reported in many studies to treat obesity and promote weight loss by reducing free radicals and lowering oxidative stress and chronic inflammation, which repair the deregulations that occur in our fat-produced metabolic adipokines.

A significant amount of research has been conducted in humans and animals on many different polyphenols that report weight-loss benefits and actions. The main mechanisms of actions reported is the reduction of oxidative stress, AGEs, and chronic inflammation, in addition to some polyphenols' ability to lower the calories in foods by blocking digestive enzymes that break down fats, sugars, and starches.

Cardiovascular Diseases

Adipokines produced in our fat cells control how we regulate our blood pressure and fluid balance, create new blood vessels, and how well our hearts contract to regulate blood flow. The direct deregulations of adipokines in fat cells created by obesity is now considered a main reason that, when we gain too much weight, we are at greater risk for developing heart problems.

In addition to fat deregulations, free radicals are particularly damaging to the cells in the heart and cardiovascular system because they are actually circulating in our bloodstream and are in constant contact. Thousands of studies report the mechanisms by which free radicals and the oxidative damage and inflammation they cause can contribute to the development of clogged arteries, high blood pressure, peripheral vascular disease, coronary artery disease, cardiomyopathy, heart failure, and cardiac arrhythmias.

Free radical damage is also the main reason people who smoke cigarettes have much higher risks for developing cardiovascular diseases. Cigarette smoke actually contains free radicals, and the chemical reactions smoke creates in the lungs generates significantly more free radicals. Chemicals used in e-cigarettes and vaping solutions are poorly studied for possible free radicals they might produce in the lungs. The recent reports of lung inflammation and lung cell death (the hallmark of free radical damage) doesn't bode well for the safety of these poorly studied chemicals going into your lungs. If you stop smoking, free radical production in your body will drop dramatically and you'll reduce the risk of free radical damage to your heart and cardiovascular system to prevent heart diseases.

Polyphenol antioxidants, including those found in chanca piedra, are the subject of a substantial body of research documenting their actions and benefits to the cardiovascular system and their ability to prevent heart diseases. Many human, animal, and in vitro studies report that polyphenols exert beneficial effects on the vascular system via the increase of antioxidant defenses and reduction of oxidative stress. These beneficial effects include lowering blood pressure, improving endothelial function, inhibiting platelet aggregation (which reduces blot clots), reducing low-density lipoprotein (LDL) cholesterol oxidation, and relieving chronic inflammation by reducing inflammatory responses. The link between polyphenol consumption and the reduction of heart disease risk is well established and widely accepted.

Neurodegenerative Diseases and Brain Disorders

Neurodegenerative disorders such as dementia, Parkinson's disease, and Alzheimer's disease represent an increasing problem in our aging societies, primarily as there is an increased prevalence of these diseases with age. These and other neurodegenerative disorders appear to be triggered by multifactorial events; however, oxidative stress and inflammation in the brain underlie most all neurodegenerative diseases and disorders. Neurons in the brain are frequent targets of oxidative stress, and the resulting cellular damage can lead to cell death and deregulation of chemical processes in the brain.

Studies looking at dietary factors and brain disorders report that regular dietary intake of polyphenol-rich foods and/or beverages has been associated with 50 percent reduction in the risk of dementia, a preservation of cognitive performance with aging, a delay in the onset of Alzheimer's disease, and a reduction in the risk of developing Parkinson's disease. Some polyphenols (including some found in chanca piedra) have been reported to reduce the neurodegeneration associated with the accumulation AGEs during normal and abnormal brain aging.

Research also suggests that some polyphenols (particularly anthocyanins) are able to cross the blood-brain barrier; thus, these polyphenol compounds are likely to be candidates for direct neuroprotective and neuromodulatory actions. Polyphenols are considered to be neuroprotective because they provide a defense against many underlying causes of neurodegenerative diseases, namely oxidative stress, neuroinflammation, protein aggregation, metal toxicity, and mitochondrial dysfunction.

There is also a growing interest in the potential of polyphenols to improve memory, learning, and general cognitive ability. Human studies suggest that polyphenols may have a positive impact on memory and depression, and there is a large body of animal behavioral research to suggest that anthocyanin polyphenols are effective at reversing age-related deficits in spatial working memory, in improving object recognition memory, and in modulating inhibitory fear conditioning.

Liver Diseases

The most leading causes of liver diseases are oxidative stress, lipid peroxidation (the oxidation of fats by free radicals), chronic inflammation, and immune response deregulations. Natural polyphenols have attracted increasing attention as potential agents for the prevention and treatment of liver diseases. Their striking capacities in relieving oxidative stress, lipid metabolism, insulin resistance, and inflammation put polyphenols in the spotlight for the therapies of liver diseases as well as for the prevention of liver diseases. Numerous studies on polyphenols and polyphenol-rich medicinal plants, including a large number of studies on chanca piedra, report the liver-protecting ability of these substances. Thousands of animal studies report that cellular-protective polyphenols can protect the liver from just about anything scientists give the animals—liver-toxic drugs, toxic doses of aspirin and alcohol, and other substances or diseases like diabetes, which are known to cause liver damage.

Age-Related Eye Diseases

Oxidative stress and inflammation play a critical role in the initiation and progression of age-related eye abnormalities such as cataracts, glaucoma, diabetic retinopathy, macular degeneration, and even the autoimmune eye disease Sjögren's syndrome. Therefore, natural plant chemicals with proven antioxidant and anti-inflammatory activities, such as carotenoids and polyphenols, could be of benefit in preventing and treating these diseases.

Antimicrobial Actions

Many polyphenols have been shown to effectively kill bacteria, viruses, and fungi in humans, just as they do in plants. This can make some polyphenols and polyphenol-rich foods natural antimicrobial agents to aid in treating infections. These antimicrobial actions are also playing a role in the friendly bacteria (and not so friendly bacteria) in our gut microbiome. The antibacterial actions of polyphenols can kill off certain types of gut bacteria, yet paradoxically, other friendly bacteria are immune and use polyphenols as a food source (prebiotic) to increase in strength and numbers. Most of the gut microbiome research with polyphenols indicates they can modulate the bacterial species in a manner to treat obesity, help maintain a healthy weight more easily, reduce intestinal inflammation, and treat or prevent chronic bowel diseases such as irritable bowel syndrome and inflammatory bowel diseases. Many polyphenols in chanca piedra have been documented with antimicrobial actions against viruses, bacteria, and fungi.

Cholesterol Modification

The majority of polyphenols play a beneficial role in the biochemical processes of how the human body processes fat in the diet. This benefit is largely attributed to the antioxidant action of polyphenols and preventing the changes in the biochemical process that occur from the actions of free radicals. The effects of free radicals can result in oxidized fat cells, causing deregulated cholesterol and triglyceride levels, the promotion of clogged arteries, and heart and vein damage, leading to high blood pressure and heart diseases. A classification of antioxidants called anthocyanins are the strongest among the polyphenols that benefit the heart and cholesterol levels.

The Polyphenols in Chanca Piedra

Chanca piedra is a particularly good example that the polyphenol profiles of medicinal plants are very different from the polyphenol profiles of common superfruits, vegetables, and beverages like coffee and red wine, which are touted for health benefits due to their high levels of polyphenols. While chanca piedra contains a handful of regular polyphenols found in many fruits and vegetables (such as gallic acid, chlorogenic acid, rutin, and quercetin), the majority of the polyphenols in chanca piedra are not found in fruits and vegetables, and you won't be getting these beneficial compounds from regular dietary sources.

Certain polyphenols are found *only* in chanca piedra, and others are found only in related medicinal *Phyllanthus* plants. These novel chemicals fall into a category of polyphenols called lignans and tannins. Chanca piedra contains quite a few lignans, and, when we digest them, these lignans regularly form bonds with other polyphenols and with other natural compounds in our bodies to form many more polyphenol metabolites and derivatives. In fact, more than 80 new polyphenols and their derivatives and metabolites were discovered in *Phyllanthus* plants between 2016 and 2018—in just two years. While the polyphenol content in plants can vary based on growing and harvesting conditions, overall, chanca piedra delivers an average of 220 to 250 milligrams of polyphenols in just 1 gram of dried whole-herb chanca piedra.

Some of chanca piedra's novel polyphenol compounds have been the subject of research to determine their pharmacological effects. A few of these chemicals have been synthesized by scientists (copied in the laboratory without using the plant) and are the subject of ongoing pharmaceutical drug company research in an effort to create new drugs. The following table highlights a few of chanca piedra's polyphenols and their effects that have been documented in research.

Compound	Documented Pharmacological Effect
Amariin	Antioxidant, hepatoprotective, radioprotective
Corilagin	Analgesic, antidiabetic, antifungal, anti-HIV, anti-inflammatory, antioxidant, antiplatelet, antitumor, antiviral, hypotensive, radioprotective, thrombolytic, vasorelaxant
Furosin	Analgesic, antioxidant, wound healing
Geraniin	Analgesic, antioxidant, anti-HIV, antimalarial, antitumor, antiviral, hepatoprotective, hypotensive, immunomodulating, radioprotective, wound healing

Hinokinin	Antioxidant, antiviral
Hypophyllanthin	Anticancer, anti-genotoxic, antitumor, antiviral, hepatoprotective, hypotensive
Isocorilagin	Antioxidant, antitumor, cholinesterase inhibitor
Lintetralin	Anti-inflammatory, antiviral
Methyl brevifolin carboxylate	Antiplatelet, anti-inflammatory, antioxidant, hypotensive
Niranthin	Analgesic, anti-inflammatory, antioxidant, anti-parasitic, antitumor, antiviral
Nirtetralin	Anti-inflammatory, antioxidant, antitumor, antiviral, hypotensive; reverses multidrug resistance
Phyllanthin	Anti-aging, anti-amnestic, antibacterial, anticancer, anti-genotoxic, antioxidant, antiviral, hypouricemic, anti-inflammatory, antileukemic, antioxidant, antitumor, cell protective, hepatoprotective, hypotensive, kidney and renal protective, immunomodulatory, reverse transcriptase inhibitor (anti-HIV)
Phyltetralin	Anti-inflammatory, antioxidant, antiviral

The polyphenols documented in chanca piedra include the following: 1-O-galloyl-2,4-dehydrohexahydroxydiphenoyl-glucopyranose, 1-galloyl-2,3-dehydrohexahydroxydiphenyl-glucose, 2,3-desmethoxy seco-isolintetralin diacetate, 2,3-desmethoxy seco-isolintetralin, 3,4-methylenedioxybenzyl-3′,4′-dimethoxybenzylbutyrolactone, 5-demethoxy-niranthin, amariin, amariinic acid, astragalin, brevifolin carboxylic acid, catechins, chlorogenic acid, corilagin, cubebin-dimethyl-ether, demethylenedioxy-niranthin, elaeocarpusin, ellagic acid, fisetin-4-O-glucoside, gallic acid, gallocatechins, geraniin, geraniinic acid, hydroxyniranthin, hypophyllanthin, isocorilagin, isolintetralin, isolintetralin, isoquercitrin, kaempferol 3-O-d-glucopyranoside, kaempferol, linnanthin, lintetralin, methyl brevifolincarboxylate, niranthin, nirphyllin, nirtetralin, niruriflavones, nirurin, niruriside, phyllamyricin D-F, phyllamyricoside A-C, phyllanthenol, phyllanthenone, phyllantheol, phyllanthin, phyllanthin, phyllanthine, phyllanthusiin A-D, phyllnirurin, phyllochrysine, phyltetralin, quercetin, quercetin-3-O-glucopyranoside, quercetol, quercitrin, repandusinic acid, rutin, seco-4-hydroxylintetralin, seco-isolariciresinol-trimethyl-ether, urinatetralin, and virgatusin.

Summary

All told, chanca piedra delivers more than 70 polyphenols, including some of the derivatives and metabolites that were created in the herb before it was harvested for use. There is simply no way to determine how many other beneficial polyphenol metabolite compounds are formed inside our bodies when we ingest chanca piedra. Many of this herb's traditional uses have been shown in studies to provide the specific medical benefits outlined in this chapter. The next two chapters will explain the actual research that has been conducted on chanca piedra. We'll first look at the research confirming its benefits to the kidneys, which indicates that, in addition to treating kidney stones, chanca piedra's kidney-protective and detoxing actions result from the actions of its many strong cellular-protective polyphenol compounds.

CHAPTER 3

Chanca Piedra's Actions on the Kidneys

One of the most notable areas of study on chanca piedra has validated its long-standing traditional use for kidney stones. There is a reason the plant was named "stone breaker"—it works well to break up kidney stones and expel them from the body. The company I founded in 1995, Raintree Nutrition, Inc., was one of the first reputable commercial sources of chanca piedra in the American herbal products market. I chose to use the Peruvian name because I was harvesting the herb in Peru. (When introducing a medicinal rainforest plant to the marketplace through my company, I generally chose to use the common name as a tribute to the country of origin from which I extracted the plant and also to highlight its local traditional uses.)

This chapter will first review the four types of kidney stones and then discuss the science and research on how chanca piedra can treat and prevent certain types. You'll learn about the significant research conducted on this treasured rainforest herb for the treatment of kidney stones, gout, cystitis, and urinary tract infections, as well as for the prevention or treatment of diabetic kidney disease and renal failure, and for its other kidney-protective benefits. I will also explain how I've used chanca piedra as a product formulator and practitioner.

The Development of Kidney Stones and the Different Types

Kidney stones affect 10 to 12 percent of the population in industrialized countries. Each year, more than half a million people go to emergency rooms for kidney stone problems. And it's usually the excruciating pain caused by the stone(s) that sends them there. Passing a kidney stone is often described as one of the most painful experiences a person can have. It is estimated that one in 10 people in the United States will have a kidney stone at some time in their lives. The prevalence of kidney stones has tripled since the 1970s, and it's not too hard to understand why. Chronic diseases such as high blood pressure, diabetes, and obesity increase the risk of kidney stones, and the epidemic rise of just these three conditions is now affecting almost half of the population.

Kidney stones actually have many causes and can affect any part of the urinary tract, from the kidneys to the bladder. Often, stones form when the urine becomes too concentrated, allowing minerals to crystallize and stick together. Basically, the main purpose of urine is to carry various wastes from our bodies, and these wastes are dissolved in the urine. When there is too much waste in too little liquid, crystals begin to form. Not drinking enough water results in dehydration, and this immediately affects the volume of liquid in the urine, concentrating it, and significantly increasing the risks of forming crystals. The crystals attract other elements, including calcium, oxalate, urate, cystine, xanthine, and phosphate, which are regular components found in urine. When these elements join and bond together, they form a solid that will get larger unless it is passed out of the body with the urine.

Diet and lifestyle can also increase the risks of developing kidney stones. Possible causes include drinking too little water, exercise levels (either too much or too little), obesity, weight-loss surgery, or eating food with too much salt or sugar. Consuming too much fructose, which is found in table sugar and high-fructose corn syrup, correlates with an increased risk of developing a kidney stone. Also, regularly eating high amounts of organ meats and shellfish can increase the risk. Infections and family genetics can also be a cause in some people.

There are basically four different types of kidney stones: cysteine stones, struvite stones, uric acid stones, and calcium stones.

Cysteine stones are caused by too much cystine. Elevated cystine levels are rare and usually have a genetic connection; therefore, cystine stones are uncommon. Struvite stones are caused by an infection and contain ammonia, which is produced by bacteria. Reoccurring urinary tract infections can increase the risk of struvite stones.

Uric acid stones are caused by too much uric acid. These are a common type of kidney stone. Foods such as red meat, organ meats, and shellfish have high concentrations of a natural chemical compound known as purines. Purines encourage the production of another chemical produced in the body called uric acid, which increases the risk of developing uric acid stones. Higher uric acid excretion leads to lower overall urine pH, which means the urine is more acidic. The high acid concentration of the urine makes it easier for uric acid stones to form. People with high-protein diets can be at greater risk for developing these types of stones.

Calcium stones are caused by calcium binding with oxalate or phosphate. Calcium stones are the most common of all types of kidney stones and are typically the result of dietary factors and hydration levels. Calcium is a normal part of a healthy diet. The kidneys usually remove excess calcium. Often the bodies of those with these stones retain too much calcium. This calcium combines with waste products like oxalate or phosphate inside the kidney to form a stone.

Calcium-oxalate stones are the most common and are formed when oxalate, a byproduct of certain foods, binds to calcium as urine is being made by the kidneys. Both oxalate and calcium are increased when the body doesn't have enough fluids (and also has too much salt). However, as confusing at it seems, people with low dairy intake in their diets are at greater risk of developing these calcium stones. Eating dairy products, which contain calcium, causes the calcium to bind with oxalate during digestion before it ever gets into the kidneys. This helps reduce the amount of oxalate available to form stones in the kidneys. Many foods contain oxalate, including many healthy foods. Those foods with the highest levels of oxalate include dark-green vegetables such as spinach, berries and cranberries, nuts, dried beans, beets, chocolate, sweet potatoes, coffee, tea, and beer. Consuming these types of foods and beverages usually isn't a problem for most as long as hydration and calcium levels are normal. Those who have already had calcium-oxalate stones are usually advised by their doctors to follow a low-oxalate diet and eliminate or reduce these high-oxalate foods.

After a stone is formed by whichever means discussed, it can either stay in the kidney or travel down the urinary tract into the ureter. Oftentimes, very small stones are flushed out of the body in the urine without causing too much pain. But stones that don't move may cause a backup of urine in the kidney, ureter, bladder, or urethra. This is what causes the pain. Also, stones are crystal-based and have sharp, uneven edges so it's much like having a cocklebur traveling around in your urinary tract, causing pain wherever it goes. The size of the stone is a major factor in whether it can be passed naturally. Stones smaller than 4 millimeters (mm) pass on their own about 80 percent of the time. They take an average of 31 days to pass. Stones that are 4 to 6 mm are more likely to require some sort of treatment, but around 60 percent pass naturally within about 45 to 60 days. Stones that are much larger usually require medical intervention to reduce their size since they're too big to fit through the urethra. The standard treatment is called extracorporeal shock wave lithotripsy, and shockwaves are used to break up the stone into much smaller pieces. However, the painful process of passing the smaller pieces is still required. Sometimes, it can take more than one treatment to break up the stones into pieces small enough to expel naturally.

The relapse rate for kidney stones is above 50 percent, which means if you've had kidney stones in the past, you're more likely to develop them again. This is typically because we all have established dietary and lifestyle patterns that we rarely change, or we have genetic factors that will never change.

Personal Experience

I first learned about chanca piedra by reading a book by Nicole Maxwell titled *Witch Doctor's Apprentice: Hunting for Medicinal Plants in the Amazon*, which was published in 1990. Nicole Maxwell was an early influencer in my life—in the 1960s, she began traveling the Amazon rainforest to study the local population's uses of their medicinal plants—and if one gutsy woman could do it, so could I! Although she was initially funded by a pharmaceutical company looking for novel plant chemicals within the richness of the undiscovered plants in the Amazon that they could turn into drugs, she was a true pioneer in cataloging the ethnobotanical uses of medicinal plants of the Amazonian rainforest. Nicole reported in her book that chanca piedra was the most respected herbal remedy in the region to treat kidney stones. She also wrote of a doctor in Nuremburg, Germany, Dr. Wolfram Wiemann, who treated over 100 kidney stone patients with chanca piedra tea and found it to be 94 percent successful in eliminating kidney stones within a week or two.

When I began my own travels in the Amazon in the mid-1990s to learn how the local people and indigenous Indian tribes used their plants as medicines and to set up harvesting of rainforest plants for my company, I found out quite quickly that Nicole Maxwell was right. Chanca piedra is a very well-known and well-respected herbal remedy that was usually one of the first remedies mentioned when I asked people in Peru about the plants they used for medicines. I also learned that calcium-oxalate kidney stones were a cultural issue in Peru's remote subsistence farming and fishing communities. One factor is that beans, which are very high in oxalate, were a main staple in their diet and were served at every meal, oftentimes, even at breakfast! Dairy products require refrigeration, and with no electricity in these remote villages, the main source of calcium in their diet was from plants. This often resulted in lower calcium levels, which led to the body storing more calcium. What's more, a lack of sanitized drinking water resulted in lower water consumption, and the heat and humidity of the climate promoted more sweating. Therefore, less than adequate hydration combined with a high-oxalate diet and higher stored calcium levels made calcium oxalate kidney stones pretty common.

Some of these remote river communities began wild-harvesting medicinal plants for my company so I made many friends and had an inside look at their culture. I learned that cultural beliefs in these remote communities also resulted in more women suffering with kidney stones than men. Many women told me they believed that sweating was "unladylike" and not attractive to their men, and they intentionally drank much less water so they didn't sweat as much. With low hydration and lots of oxalate in the diet, kidney stones were a common "woman's aliment." For this reason, chanca piedra was often the first medicinal plant women referred to; they used it often to either treat or prevent kidney stones.

When I first launched chanca piedra in my company retail product line, it was sold in capsules, a liquid extract, and in a bulk powder for making tea. After much research on the active chemicals in the herb, I chose to manufacture a water/glycerin extract of chanca piedra. I discovered most of chanca piedra's active chemicals were water soluble and some were very delicate—using alcohol to make a tincture extract wasn't necessary and would have resulted in the loss of some of the herb's beneficial and active chemicals, including some important but delicate polyphenols.

I also used chanca piedra as a main ingredient in three multi-herb formulas I created for kidney health that were sold only to practitioners. Amazon Kidney Support was formulated specifically for kidney stones, Amazon Urinary Support was formulated for urinary tract infections, and Amazon KDY-CL was formulated for cleansing and detoxing the kidneys as well as kidney regeneration and protection during diabetes and dialysis. I chose to produce formulas for the alternative health practitioner's market because what I could legally say about a retail product to a trained health practitioner was much more substantial than what I could share with the public. I educated licensed practitioners on the actions and benefits of my formulas based on the clinical and published research on their plant ingredients. As practitioners used these formulas for their patients with success, word of mouth spread from patients to friends and relatives, and increasing numbers of people learned about these effective rainforest medicinal plants and formulas and what to use them for.

The chanca piedra products and formulas I developed were some of the most popular in the product line. Effective products almost sell themselves. Sales were generated, and they increased quickly, based solely on their effectiveness. Retail customers buying just chanca piedra had good results treating their kidney stones and gout (more on that later) and spread the word about their effectiveness in eliminating small- to medium-sized calcium or uric acid stones, usually within two weeks or less. Those using the multi-herb formula had quicker results (some within just a couple of days), and it worked better for uric acid stones. These products generated many testimonials (which couldn't be legally published or used to promote products) on their ability to almost immediately help relieve the intense pain associated with kidney stones and gout, which was obviously much appreciated. The Urinary Support formula had quite a large practitioner following and even among some conventional urologists who sold the formula in their offices for hard-to-treat reoccurring urinary tract infections that were resistant to normal antibiotic therapy. See the resource section for more information on these formulas and how you can prepare them for yourself.

A large amount of research has been conducted on chanca piedra since I first created these formulas, and much of it explains why chanca piedra and these three formulas worked so well to provide dramatic results. The rest of this chapter will focus on the research on chanca piedra's effects on the kidneys.

How Chanca Piedra Treats Kidney Stones

When all the research conducted on chanca piedra's ability to treat active kidney stones is reviewed, the following mechanism of actions have been demonstrated in animals and humans:

- Chanca piedra has diuretic actions (increases urination), which may be helpful to flush small stones out of the kidney and urinary tract more quickly and efficiently.

- ❑ Chanca piedra has antispasmodic and smooth-muscle relaxation actions that relax the smooth muscles in the bladder and urethra to promote easier and smoother expulsion of stones. Novel alkaloids in chanca piedra demonstrated smooth-muscle relaxation specific to the urinary and biliary tract.
- ❑ Chanca piedra has a direct action on the structure of stones and can reduce the crystallization on the outer surface of the stone. This reduces the sharp edges, makes the stones smaller in size, and helps stones to glide more smoothly (and with less pain) through the urinary tract during expulsion.
- ❑ Chanca piedra can chemically interfere with crystal formation and growth. This helps prevent existing stones from growing larger and is also useful for preventing new stones from forming for preventative purposes.
- ❑ Chanca piedra lowers uric acid, calcium, and oxalate levels in the kidneys. This removes the building blocks of stones where they are formed, stops existing stones from increasing in size, and prevents new stones from forming.
- ❑ Chanca piedra promotes the increase of several anti-stone chemicals produced in our bodies (including magnesium, potassium, citrate, and others) to increase natural processes that help prevent the formation of stones.
- ❑ Chanca piedra has pain-relieving actions (comparable to a pain drug called tramadol), which helps relieve kidney stone pain while the plant is working to expel stones.

- While many natural compounds in chanca piedra are providing beneficial actions, the novel lignan polyphenols—phyllanthin, hypophyllanthin, and phyltetralin—have demonstrated specific actions to lower uric acid, oxalate, and calcium levels in research on animals. Other novel triterpenes in the plant were also discovered to help reduce crystallization and reduce the size of stones.

Despite its "stone breaker" or "shatter stone" name, chanca piedra is not capable of breaking large stones into smaller pieces. It can reduce the size of stones by a several millimeters by acting on the surface of a stone, but it cannot break up very large stones like shock-wave treatment can. For that reason, researchers report that chanca piedra's highest and best use is for small- to medium-size stones, and it is beneficial to combine with shock-wave therapy to help expel the smaller pieces of a large stone that shock-wave therapy breaks up.

One of the first research studies to confirm chanca piedra's traditional use for kidney stones was published in 1990 by the Paulista School of Medicine in São Paulo, Brazil. They gave humans and rats a simple tea of chanca piedra for one to three months and reported that it promoted the elimination of stones. They also reported a significant increase in urine output as well as sodium and creatine excretion. Subsequently, the medical school educated new doctors about the ability to treat kidney stones with this natural remedy, and now it is found in many pharmacies throughout Brazil. Previously (in the mid-1980s), the antispasmodic activity of chanca piedra was reported. This led the Brazilian researchers to surmise that "smooth muscle relaxation within the urinary or biliary tract probably facilitates the expulsion of kidney or bladder calculi." Other researchers in India had already reported chanca piedra's smooth-muscle relaxant properties in earlier studies published in the 1950s.

In a 1999 test-tube study, a chanca piedra extract exhibited the ability to block the formation of calcium-oxalate crystals, which indicates that it might be a useful preventative aid for people with a history of kidney stones. In 2002, researchers seeded the bladders of rats with calcium-oxalate crystals and treated them for 42 days with a chanca piedra tea. Their results indicated that chanca piedra strongly inhibited the growth and number of stones formed compared to the control group. Several of the animals even passed the stones that did form. In 2003, scientists again confirmed that chanca piedra could help prevent the formation of kidney stones; they stated "that it may interfere with the early stages of stone formation and may represent an alternative form of treatment and/or prevention of urolithiasis."

Other research continues to support that chanca piedra is a great natural remedy to treat and prevent kidney stones. A double-blind placebo human study in 2004 reported that chanca piedra reduced urinary calcium levels, which would be helpful in reducing stone formation. In 2006, a Brazilian study with rats reported that chanca piedra was able to modify the shape and texture of stones to a smoother and probably more fragile form, which could contribute to elimination and/or dissolution of stones. Italian researchers at a university medical hospital followed 150 kidney stone patients following traditional shock-wave therapy to break up large kidney stones with half taking chanca piedra after treatment to help expel the stones and prevent new ones. Their 2006 research paper reported that for those with lower calcium stones (56 patients), the stone-free rate was 93.7 percent in the chanca piedra group and 70.8 percent in the control group. Concerning the chanca piedra treatment, they reported, "Its efficacy and the absolute lack of side effects make this therapy suitable to improve overall outcomes after extracorporeal shock wave lithotripsy for lower pole stones."

Doctors in Romania conducted another human study in 2019. They gave a low dosage of a chanca piedra extract (450 milligrams daily) to 40 patients with stones ranging from 2 to 14 millimeters in size. At the end of three months, 40 percent were stone free, 21.7 percent had a reduced size of stones, and 38 percent were unchanged. The average shrinkage of stones was by 1.7 millimeters. The product they used in the study was extracted in alcohol and then spray dried; it might have not extracted all of chanca piedra's delicate water-soluble active chemicals. The results they reported were not as effective as prior studies utilizing just a water extract or tea of the plant. This was a significant issue in most of the research on different extractions methods used in the hepatitis research that will be discussed later.

Also, in many of these kidney stone studies (and others), researchers reported that chanca piedra has a diuretic effect and significantly increases urination. A study in 2018 specifically studied this diuretic effect and reported that it almost doubled the amount of urination in rats. Another 2018 study on 56 human patients with kidney stones performed in Brazil confirmed the same diuretic action and reported that chanca piedra reduced the size of the stones, as well as significantly reduced urinary uric acid and oxalate levels in just 24 hours. At the end of the study, these researchers reported that uric acid, oxalate, calcium, and citrate levels normalized in all patients taking chanca piedra.

All in all, chanca piedra has been the subject of more than 15 human and animal studies and even more test-tube research studies on how it treats and prevents kidney stones. None of the research reported any toxicity or significant side effects, and chanca piedra was well tolerated. See the reference section for a listing of the research performed on chanca piedra's benefits and actions on kidney stones.

A Naturopathic Protocol for Kidney Stones

Most find that chanca piedra can help pass a stone in a week or less (depending on the size of the stone, with larger stones taking longer). It also works almost immediately to help relieve the excruciating pain that anyone with a kidney stone can describe quite well (more on chanca piedra's pain-relieving actions are discussed in the next chapter). The studies on chanca piedra reveal that it does works at low dosages, but it takes longer. The safety of chanca piedra is excellent, even in high dosages; therefore, I've never recommended low dosages. My clients with stones wanted fast results, and higher dosages deliver that.

If cost is an issue, I recommend that people use a whole-herb powder of chanca piedra and prepare it as a tea: 1 teaspoon of powder per one cup of water. Place a teaspoon of powder in a mug and pour boiling water into the cup. Stir, cover the mug, and allow it to steep for 10 minutes. The powder will settle to the bottom of the cup, and you can drink the tea off the top without straining. Two cups of tea daily are recommended until the stone passes. Many find capsules are easier or they don't much like the slightly bitter, grassy taste of the tea. Dosages for capsules are three 500-milligram capsules of chanca piedra whole herb three times daily. If you weigh more than 180 pounds, take four 500-milligram capsules, three times daily. Drink at least 2 quarts of water daily (even more if you can) and reduce your salt intake. Also, see the cautions and contraindications listed in chapter 5 if you have diabetes or hypertension or if you are currently taking prescription drugs.

If you have a kidney stone, you're more likely to develop more stones in the future. For prevention purposes, review your dietary habits to determine the amount of high-oxalate foods you eat regularly. Either reduce the amount of those foods in your diet, consume them in combination with dairy products, or do both. The calcium in dairy products will bind with the oxalate during digestion and prevent high oxalate levels in your kidneys. This does *not* work with calcium supplements. Always make sure your water intake is adequate and you stay hydrated. Also, you should have, at a minimum, the RDA (preferably twice the RDA) of magnesium and vitamin B6 either from your diet or from supplements—both have shown in research to help prevent the formation of stones. Take chanca piedra once weekly, either as a tea or in capsules at the same dosages previously mentioned. Since chanca piedra can lower oxalate and uric acid levels in the kidneys quickly with a single dosage, taking it once a week can help flush these stone-forming chemicals out of the kidneys and reduce the risks of crystals forming.

The key to preventing stones is to stop crystals from forming and, if they do, to expel them while they are small, rather than allowing them to grow to a much larger size that requires medical intervention.

Chanca piedra has been used for kidney stones for more than 1,000 years in the countries where it grows naturally. That human and animal studies now confirm this important traditional use is not surprising, and hopefully this research will encourage more Americans to use chanca piedra for the treatment and prevention of kidney stones. Regardless of any published research, the local population of the Amazon rainforest will continue to use it as they always have as an effective herbal remedy and as their first line of therapy for kidney stones.

Treatment and Prevention of Gout

Chanca piedra can also be a quick and effective remedy for another extremely painful condition—gout. Gout is caused by too much uric acid in body. Gout is actually a type of arthritis and occurs when excess uric acid crystalizes and deposits in the joints, causing pain and inflammation. Much of the kidney stone research reports that chanca piedra can lower uric acid levels quickly and effectively and in as little as 24 hours. Since chanca piedra also prevents uric acid from forming crystals and has a direct effect to dissolve uric crystals already formed, the plant's ability to treat gout is pretty clear. Chanca piedra's pain-relieving actions are also beneficial to immediately relieve the pain of gout as well.

The enzyme-inhibitor actions of several polyphenols

in chanca piedra may be playing a significant role in how the plant reduces uric acid. One very well-known enzyme we produce in our bodies is called xanthine oxidase (XO). This enzyme generates reactive oxygen species (ROS), and it is required for the body to manufacture uric acid. Chanca piedra (and several tested polyphenols that are in chanca piedra) has shown in research to inhibit XO, which results in lower amounts of uric acid. Also, the plant's antioxidant actions may prevent the oxidation of another enzyme that must be oxidized to produce uric acid. This will also result in less uric acid.

Chanca piedra has always been the first remedy I've recommended for the treatment and prevention of gout, and over twenty years, it has rarely failed me for this purpose. Using it with my own clients and training many practitioners about chanca piedra's effectiveness for gout have resulted in many testimonials and many more people now know just how effective it is.

The naturopathic protocol for treating and preventing gout are the same dosages previously mentioned for kidney stones. In addition, I've also educated my clients about the benefits of vitamin C for the prevention of gout. Several human studies report that higher dosages of vitamin C (500 milligrams or more daily) can significantly lower uric acid levels and treat the condition, while other studies report lower dosages (100 to 300 milligrams daily) are beneficial in preventing future gout attacks. One study followed 46,994 healthy men over 20 years to see if vitamin C intake was linked to developing gout. Interestingly, their research revealed that people who took a vitamin C supplement had a 44 percent lower gout risk.

Chronic Kidney Disease and Kidney Protective Actions

Chronic kidney disease (CKD) is a debilitating condition with various causal factors, culminating in end-stage renal disease, requiring dialysis or kidney transplantation. The progression of CKD is closely associated with systemic inflammation and oxidative stress, which are responsible for the manifestation of numerous complications such as malnutrition, atherosclerosis, coronary artery calcification, heart failure, anemia, and mineral and bone disorders, as well as increased risks of heart attacks.

The main causes of CKD are high blood pressure and diabetes, but it can also be caused by immune-mediated diseases, glomerulonephritis (inflammation of the kidneys), tubulointerstitial disease, prescription drugs (especially chemotherapy and immunosuppressant drugs), and hereditary kidney diseases. Other risk factors for developing CKD include heart disease, obesity, a family history of CKD, past damage to the kidneys, and older age. Approximately 15 percent of U.S. adults—37 million people—are estimated to have CKD, and it's estimated that 38 percent of Americans over age 65 have CKD. Almost half of those who have CKD also have diabetes and/or cardiovascular disease. The alarming increases in the rates of obesity, diabetes, and high blood pressure we've seen over the last 10 years has contributed to the rise of CKD cases over the same period.

As discussed in the previous chapter, the causal link between obesity, diabetes, high blood pressure, and heart disease is elevated levels of chronic inflammation and oxidative stress, which promote the progression of all these diseases. Diabetes and obesity significantly increase free radical production, and the resulting oxidative stress, cellular damage, and chronic inflammation can be one of CKD's main causes. For this reason, oxidative stress has become an important diagnostic and prognostic factor and is a target for CKD prevention and treatment. High levels of oxidative stress have already been found in the early stages of CKD, which increase in parallel with the progression to end-stage renal disease and is further exacerbated in dialysis patients. In fact, dialysis has been shown to increase oxidative processes, leading to an increase in oxidative stress.

In the kidneys, reactive oxygen species (ROS) are naturally produced by the mitochondria of kidney cells. If our built-in antioxidant system falters or becomes overwhelmed fighting the much higher levels of ROS in diabetes or obesity, it can immediately affect the ability of our natural antioxidants to keep these kidney cell–generated ROS under control, and cellular damage results. Excessive ROS production that cannot be neutralized by our built-in antioxidant system causes cell damage to proteins, nucleic acids, and lipids, and also affects cellular and enzyme-inhibiting activity. In addition, during CKD, there is a considerable increase in oxidative stress due to uremic toxins, substances that interact negatively with biological functions. The kidneys are responsible for flushing out waste, toxins, and other substances from the body. When kidney function declines as CKD progresses, the ability to flush these toxins declines, and these substances can accumulate in urine, kidney tissues, and cells. The damage these toxins cause create more free radicals and more inflammation.

Doctors have long known that oxidative stress and chronic inflammation are both a cause and significant factor in the progression of CKD. The main problem is that there are no effective drugs available for doctors to prescribe that address chronic inflammation and oxidative stress. The use of statin drugs and angiotensin-converting enzyme (ACE) inhibitors, as well as angiotensin II type 1 (AT1) blockers, have been shown to exert some anti-inflammatory effects, although research indicates they are not effective for dialysis patients. Our current supply of anti-inflammatory drugs were created for short-term treatment of acute inflammation rather than long-term chronic inflammation. Only two antioxidant drugs are available, but they are rarely prescribed due to significant side effects.

The huge amount of interest and research on polyphenols has, in large part, been stimulated by these natural compound's ability to effectively treat chronic inflammation and oxidative stress. Numerous studies have shown the possibility of using polyphenol compounds, including those found in chanca piedra, with anti-inflammatory and antioxidant activities in the treatment of CKD within all this polyphenol research. Unfortunately, these natural compounds cannot be patented and turned into new drugs, and research dollars just aren't available to conduct large, long-term human clinical trials on these natural polyphenols, which are required for the mainstream medical community to embrace them as new therapies. Despite the involvement of oxidative stress, antioxidant therapies have not become a standard of care in CKD patients to date, and until these types of clinical trials are conducted on natural antioxidants, it simply won't be. That leaves it up to patients to do their own research and to find nutritional therapies that will lower their free radical levels and reduce oxidative stress and chronic inflammation on their own.

Chanca piedra contains a significant amount of polyphenols with a proven ability to reduce free radicals, reduce oxidative stress, and relieve chronic inflammation. More information on the antioxidant and anti-inflammatory actions of chanca piedra is found in the next chapter. This antioxidant research also reveals that the antioxidants in chanca piedra also provide effective cellular protective actions.

Several research studies report that chanca piedra can help protect the kidneys with the actions of these cellular-protective antioxidants. Diabetes has a well-known negative effect on the kidneys, which, over time, can result in kidney damage, leading to dialysis. In an animal study in 2017, chanca piedra protected the kidneys of diabetic rats from the normal damage the disease has on the kidneys and preserved near normal kidney function by preventing oxidative stress, inflammation, fibrosis, and cell death while enhancing and encouraging the growth of new kidney cells. An earlier test-tube study in 2014 reported much of these same effects.

In other research published in 2014, Brazilian researchers gave a chanca piedra water and alcohol extract to rats that were given a chemotherapy drug, which is known to have a damaging effect on the bladder and urinary tract (as well as the liver). They reported that chanca piedra protected these organs from the usual damage, including the normal pain, inflammation, and bleeding that occurs in the bladder. These researchers suggested that chanca piedra might prove useful as an adjunctive therapy to avoid the collateral damage this chemotherapy drug causes. All three of these studies reported that the strong cellular-protective polyphenol antioxidants in chanca piedra were largely responsible for these protective effects. Researchers in Nigeria reported similar results in 2008 for *Phyllanthus amarus,* which is closely related to *Phyllanthus niruri* and has a very similar chemistry. They reported that the herb effectively protected rats from acetaminophen- and gentamicin-induced kidney damage. They also related these kidney-protective abilities to the plant's inherent antioxidant and free radical–scavenging compounds, which it shares with chanca piedra.

More than 70 studies have been published on the cellular-protective actions these antioxidant polyphenols have on the liver in a similar fashion. The research on this beneficial action is also explained in the next chapter. For whatever reason, researchers seemed to be more focused on liver protection than kidney protection over the last 10 years; therefore, many more studies were conducted on chanca piedra's liver-protective actions than just the few studies discussed with regard to the kidneys and I'm sure the same results would be found if more studies were conducted on the plant's ability to protect the kidneys.

The naturopathic protocol I've long used for CKD was the multi-herb formula I created with chanca piedra, Amazon KDY-CL. More information about the formula and how to make it yourself is in the resources section. To use chanca piedra alone, take three 500-milligram capsules twice daily for mild to moderate CKD. If you weigh more than 185 pounds, take four 500-milligram capsules twice daily. If you have advanced CKD and are already on dialysis, take three

500-milligram capsules, three times daily. Using the powder to make a tea is suitable as well. Use 1 teaspoon of chanca piedra powder in a cup of boiling water and prepare it as described earlier. Drink one or two cups daily depending on the severity and stage of CKD. If you are already on dialysis, drink two cups daily. If you've been instructed to reduce fluid intake, take capsules instead of drinking a tea. Also, see the cautions and contraindications listed in chapter 6 if you have diabetes, hypertension, or are currently taking prescription drugs.

Urinary Tract Infections

Chanca piedra has been traditionally used in herbal medicine systems around the world to treat urinary tract infections (UTIs). You'll learn in the next chapter about the research that confirms chanca piedra has antibacterial actions. Common bacteria continue to mutate to create a defensive mechanism against our gold-standard antibiotics. There are now five different strains of *E. coli* that commonly cause UTIs. Researchers in Nigeria tested chanca piedra (as well as *Phyllanthus amarus*) against all five strains *in vitro* (in a test tube) and reported both had antibacterial actions against all strains, but chanca piedra was much stronger than its closely related species *Phyllanthus amarus*.

The naturopathic protocol I've long used for UTIs was the multi-herb formula called Amazon Urinary Support. It combined chanca piedra with several other rainforest plants with strong antibacterial and antifungal actions and was specifically formulated for UTIs. I learned early on that many long-standing chronic UTIs (as well as prostate infections) treated with repeated courses of antibiotics could often cause a hidden fungal infection in the urinary tract. There are lots of friendly bacteria in our guts and genitourinary tract whose roles are to keep candida and fungus in check, which can be wiped out by prescription antibiotics. If the infection reoccurred after 30 to 45 days following a course of antibiotics, I concluded it could be a fungal infection rather than a bacterial infection. The benefit of using multiple plants with multiple actions against bacteria, candida, and fungus resulted in the urinary formula being effective for the majority of UTIs, regardless of which microbe was the culprit or even needing to know which microbe was the problem. In addition, other plants in the formula were effective against antibiotic-resistant strains of bacteria, and using a formula containing many different antibacterial natural compounds prevents bacteria from mutating the way it can with a single-chemical compound to avoid eradication. More information on the urinary support formula and how to prepare it and use it is in the resource section.

To use just chanca piedra for UTIs, take three or four 500-milligram capsules (take four capsules if you weigh more than 185 pounds) three times daily, or two cups of chanca piedra tea twice daily prepared as previously discussed.

Summary

I have used chanca piedra for my clients and in formulating herbal remedies for more than 20 years. When I need to address kidney or liver issues (more on that in the next chapter), it's always the first herbal remedy I choose. And, as a single herbal remedy for kidney stones, I don't know of anything better or faster. One of my granddaughters has reoccurring stones, and as soon as the kidney pain starts, she drinks a cup of chanca piedra tea. Usually the stone passes by the second or third cup. She's learned that it's much easier to pass stones while they are much smaller, and chanca piedra works perfectly for this purpose. In all the years I've used chanca piedra, there were no problems with tolerability or side effects, and the human studies conducted on the herb report the same safety and tolerability profile of this effective herbal remedy.

CHAPTER 4

Chanca Piedra and Emerging Infectious Diseases

It has long been known by doctors and scientists that bacteria, viruses, parasites, fungi, and other disease-causing microorganisms can readily develop defense mechanisms against our prescription drugs and become drug resistant. Many have already, as is readily apparent in the news today. The common staph bacteria (*Staphylococcus*) has gone through so many mutations over the last 30 years that many different strains have evolved that are now completely resistant to the eight major antibiotic drugs that were once effective against it. There are also at least five new strains of malaria that are now completely resistant to our gold-standard antimalarial drugs. The hepatitis virus has continued to mutate into new types and subtypes, and our antiviral drugs are largely ineffective. Could plants hold the answer? Very possibly!

Are Rainforest Plants the Answer?

The rainforests of the world are, and will continue to be, of the most utmost importance and one of the main areas where the search for new antimicrobial drugs will likely take place. Rainforests hold the highest biodiversity and sheer number of novel chemicals on the planet. Acre for acre, there are more species of plants, animals, insects, and even microbial species such as bacteria, fungi, and viruses than anywhere on earth. It is estimated that one-half of all species on earth are found in tropical rainforests.

In the species-rich rainforest, there are many species of fungi, mold, bacteria, viruses, parasites, and even insects that attack and kill plants. It is of little wonder that rainforest plants contain so many potent and active plant chemicals—they are in a constant battle for survival in an environment literally teeming with life that is constantly evolving. From the soil-borne root-rot (a virus) that attacks tender herbaceous plants, to the fungi and mold smothering the life out of huge canopy trees or even the incredible amount of insects devouring any defenseless leaf in the forest . . . rainforest plants have learned to adapt, create chemical defenses against attack and to survive.

Within this rich arsenal of defensive chemicals, many rainforest plants have been tested with antibacterial, antiviral, anti-fungal, anti-parasitic, anti-mold and insecticidal chemicals with potent actions. It is likely that within these diverse chemicals created to protect the plants from disease, at least a handful of highly active chemicals can and will be harvested and put to the use of protecting humans and animals from the same types of disease-causing organisms. Chanca piedra has been targeted within this search for active chemicals capable of killing microorganisms and research is ongoing on several active chanca piedra natural compounds.

A very interesting emerging concept is that many disease-causing microorganisms can pretty easily adapt and mutate to become resistant to a single chemical, but it would be much harder and take much more time for it to create a defense mechanism against numerous different chemicals simultaneously. Unlike a single-chemical drug, a single medicinal plant can contain up to 300 different chemicals or more, many of which have active biological properties. Could this hold the answer? Very possibly! For example, a rainforest Indian shaman's "dysentery remedy" was evaluated years back by scientists. It was a crude plant extract that contained seven plants.

Now, one must remember, a dysentery diagnosis in the Amazon could be attributed to any number of different bacteria, amoebas, and even parasites in contaminated communal food and water supplies. An Indian shaman can't send blood or stool samples to a laboratory to find out which specific organism is causing the dysentery in his village, but he must still select the appropriate plants to treat his patients. Maybe this is why a shaman usually selects a handful of plants (about four to seven) rather than just one to brew into a plant-based remedy.

When the seven different plants in the dysentery remedy were analyzed, at least twelve different known antibacterial chemicals, five anti-amoebic chemicals, and seven antiparasitic chemicals were found between all the plants in the shaman's formula. Of the 12 different antibacterial chemicals in the extract, there were at least five different biological pathways of action that the plant chemicals possessed to kill bacteria. Based on just the chemical content of the plant extract and the number of different dysentery-causing microbes that were susceptible to these chemicals, the shaman didn't really need to know which microorganism was the culprit in what mainstream medicine would call his "shotgun" approach. However, his shotgun was loaded with a thousand or more individual plant chemicals that had at least 31 active chemicals, which hit the top 10 or so main microbes that might cause dysentery—and it was effective. Imagine if your conventional practitioner sent you home with 31 prescriptions . . . you'd think the doctor was crazy!

But let's go back to that interesting concept. If this particular dysentery microbe was an easily mutating bacteria like *Staphylococcus* or *E. coli*, how likely would it be that this one organism could survive long enough to create a defense against 12 different antibacterial chemicals coming at it and in at least five different ways simultaneously? Not very likely. That's why, sometimes, plants really can be better than drugs. These drug-resistant strains of bacteria are certainly more prevalent in first-world nations, which regularly employ single-chemical antibiotics, than in poor tropical countries where mainly plant-based remedies are used. Maybe it will take a broadly scattering "shotgun" to fight these tricky and quickly mutating organisms, instead of single-chemical bullet.

As more of our gold-standard single-bullet drugs become less effective against newly developing strains of drug-resistant bacteria, viruses, fungi, and parasites, we are seeing more interest and research on medicinal plants, herbal-based drugs, and traditional remedies. Much of this research is taking place in the rainforests of the world. Many rainforest plants, including chanca piedra, have been identified through laboratory research to possess antimicrobial actions. For more information about antimicrobial rainforest plants and the research conducted on them, see the online Tropical Plant Database at www.rain-tree.com, or they can be found in my book *The Healing Power of Rainforest Herbs*.

Before we look at the large body of research on which bacteria, viruses, and other microbes that chanca piedra has been documented to kill, we need to look at an important aspect chanca piedra provides to help fight infectious diseases—supporting our immune system to effectively fight infections as it was designed to do. Our immune system is really our first line of defense against infectious diseases. As discussed in chapter 2, many polyphenols can modulate the immune system's production of various pro-inflammatory chemicals. This type of immunomodulation results in reducing inflammation. Chanca piedra has quite a few of these types of polyphenols, and the herb's ability to modulate the immune system is attributed, in part, to these well-known natural compounds and their well-documented actions. However, chanca piedra has some novel chemicals as well that have been documented with the ability to increase the immune system's ability to fight bacterial and viral infections.

Immune-Modulation Actions

Chanca piedra has been the subject of a great deal of research, including human clinical trials, on its ability to modulate the immune system. This research has revealed that chanca piedra can reduce the levels of pro-inflammatory chemicals (called cytokines) produced by the immune system to relieve inflammation, while at the same time, increase other immune cells that fight infections and create a natural immunity to various infections. In all the research, two main novel compounds have surfaced as at least two of the main immunomodulatory compounds: phyllanthin and hypophyllanthin. These two chemicals have been extracted from chanca piedra and tested individually for their immunomodulation benefits.

One of the latest studies in this area of research was published in 2019. Researchers in China studied these two chemicals in an asthmatic rodent model. Asthma is a chronic immunoinflammatory disorder so it's easy to test a drug or plant compound's ability to modulate the immune system to reduce inflammation in asthmatic animals. They reported that both novel chemicals immediately and significantly reduced the pro-inflammatory immune response and suggested that phyllanthin and hypophyllanthin may be a new therapeutic approach for the management of asthma.

The use of chanca piedra as an as an immunomodulator has been scientifically studied and evaluated in various human clinical trials for the treatment of chronic hepatitis B, pulmonary tuberculosis, candida vaginitis, Hanson's disease (leprosy), as well as a herpes virus called *Varicella zoster* infection (chicken pox) in children. Some of these studies were randomized, double-blind, placebo-controlled clinical studies, which are the gold standard in human research. In such diseases, a good immune system response is crucial to the treatment success and eradication of the pathogens. In these clinical studies, chanca piedra was proven for its capacity to modulate and activate the immune system to help fight these infections as well as create immunity cells to help protect against future infection.

In fact, it was also noted in several of these human studies that immune cells responsible for immunity were also increased, and those taking chanca piedra for their infections had no relapses or secondary infections and had higher levels of antigens (cells responsible for immunity). All patients studied with these infections mounted a better immune response and recovered more quickly. The small trial on leprosy patients led researchers to surmise that its strong and immediate immunity response might be helpful as a preventative or anti-infection remedy to protect caregivers of this devastating disease.

Much of this clinical research was conducted in Indonesia and Malaysia where chanca piedra is sold as an herbal drug. Their research confirms the enhancing activities and function of immune system components, both humoral and cellular immunities, that chanca piedra provides. There are also numerous *in vitro* and animal studies reporting potential benefits of the immunomodulatory properties of chanca piedra.

Specifically, the human and animal research reports that chanca piedra activates immune cells (neutrophils, macrophages/monocytes, and T and B lymphocytes). The activation of the phagocytic process (the ability of immune cells to kill invading pathogens) by neutrophils suggests a quicker eradication process of invading bacteria, viruses, or fungi, and their clearance out of the body. Additionally, modulation of cytokine expression and secretion (IFN-γ, TNF-α, IL-4, IL-6, IL-12, L-10) observed in the clinical studies provide a strong indication that chanca piedra may also influence the defense reactions of the body against foreign pathogens involving cellular immune function.

The culmination of all this research indicates that chanca

piedra is a good herbal remedy to support the immune system and help the immune system fight against infections without overstimulation of inflammation that the innate immune system usually employs to fight these infections. Once again, the human clinical research conducted on these abilities reported that chanca piedra was well tolerated, and no signs of toxicity or side effects were reported, even when used for children as young as three years old who had chicken pox. A list of the research on chanca piedra's immunomodulation actions is found in the references section.

Recovering from viral infections especially is mostly dependent on the effectiveness of the immune system to kill viral cells naturally, and chanca piedra has surfaced an important remedy to boost immune function during viral infection. The main reason is that we have few effective antiviral drugs for many types of viruses. It's hard for pharmaceutical companies to justify the cost of developing new antiviral drugs since, by the time a drug is approved, the virus may have mutated enough that their new drug is no longer effective against it. Many viruses will run their course of infection and resolve themselves if immune function is normal. However, in addition to kidney stones, chanca piedra is renowned for its ability to actually kill various types of viruses such as hepatitis B and C, HIV, various herpes viruses, and even flu viruses. In much of the antiviral research, doctors and scientists often reported an increased immune response, which was at least partially responsible for chanca piedra's benefits to treat viral infections. However, chanca piedra can actually kill viruses or prevent them from growing and spreading as well. This body of antiviral research will be discussed next.

Antiviral Actions

Chanca piedra was first reported to have antiviral actions against hepatitis B in the mid 1980s, and it has been widely studied around the world for its antiviral actions ever since. Over 20 clinical studies have been published to date about these effects, and the results have been inconsistent and confusing (unless thoroughly evaluated).

Hepatitis is enough of a worldwide concern to merit sifting through the disparate studies. Hepatitis B infection (HBV) is the leading cause of liver cancer worldwide—which is considered almost 100 percent fatal. Carriers of HBV are 200 times more likely to develop liver cancer decades after initial infection. Many people who contract HBV become chronic (and, often, asymptomatic) carriers of the disease while still being contagious to others. HBV is reported to be 100 times more infectious than HIV and, like HIV, is transmitted through blood transfusions, needles, sexual contact, and in utero (from mother to child in the womb). Statistics on HBV are staggering: one out of every 250 Americans are HBV carriers! The Centers for Disease Control and Prevention (CDC) estimates that 200,000 new U.S. cases of HBV infection per year are added to the current estimate of 1 million carriers in the United States (and an estimated 300 million worldwide). The CDC also reports that in the United States 3,000 to 4,000 annual deaths from cirrhosis and 1,000 deaths from liver cancer are HBV-related. So when Dr. Baruch Blumberg reported that chanca piedra could clear up the chronic carrier state of hepatitis B in 1988, it was a big deal. Dr. Blumberg was the winner of the 1963 Nobel Prize for discovering the HBV antigen in the first place. This led to the discovery that HBV was the primary cause of liver cancer and initiated the development of HBV vaccines.

Most of Blumberg's early research was carried out in India in collaboration with an Indian research group. Their first human study reported that a water extract of *Phyllanthus amarus* cleared the HBV surface antigen from 22 of 37 chronic HBV patients in only 30 days (and they continued to test negative for nine months, at which time the report was published). This same group had published several earlier *in vitro* studies as well as animal (woodchuck) studies. (Woodchucks respond to chronic HBV infection in much the same manner as do humans, which is why they are chosen for such research.) All reported similar and effective anti-HBV effects. By that time, Blumberg was employed with the Fox Chase Cancer Center in Philadelphia; he, Fox Chase, and the Indian researchers filed two patents on the plant's ability to treat HBV and its antiviral properties in 1985 and 1988 (now calling the plant *Phyllanthus niruri* or chanca piedra). The first patent was specific to HBV; the second stated that the plant's antiviral properties were achieved in part through a strong inhibition of reverse transcriptase (chemicals necessary for many types of viruses to grow), which made it possible to treat such retroviruses as HIV as well as sarcoma and leukemia viruses.

It was also during this time that the group developed a new and "better" extraction process. This process involved multiple complicated extractions in which the plant was first soaked in cold water, then the resulting fluid was extracted first in hexane, then in benzene, then in methanol, and then back into water. Their documentation revealed, however, that they didn't know specifically what the active chemicals were in the final extract that were providing the antiviral effects! While it was certainly a complicated and patentable process, much of the subsequent published research by this group throughout the 1990s using this new patented "water extract" conflicted with their earlier studies and was not as effective in the *in vivo* research for HBV. This caused much confusion as to whether chanca piedra (*Phyllanthus niruri* or *Phyllanthus amarus*) was an effective treatment or not. To add to the confusion, in 1994, a New Zealand research group prepared a chemically altered extract of *Phyllanthus amarus* that was standardized to the geraniin chemical content (the chemical documented with analgesic and hypotensive properties). They started a double-blind HBV human trial, later discontinued it due to lack of response, and published another negative result study.

Meanwhile, a separate research group in China (where HBV is wide spread) working with a straight water extract and/or herb powder published two positive studies showing good results with human HBV patients in 1994 and 1995. Their second study suggested that different results were obtained through different *Phyllanthus* species of plants used (and that yet another species, *Phyllanthus urinaria,* provided the best anti-HBV results). Chinese researchers published a 2001 study that compared 30 chronic HBV patients taking a chanca piedra extract to 25 patients taking interferon (the leading conventional drug at the time that was used for HBV) for three months. Both treatments showed an equal effectiveness of 83 percent, but the chanca piedra group rated significantly higher in the normalization of liver enzymes and recovery of liver function than the interferon-treated group. They published yet another study in 2003 that attributed the anti-HVB effects mainly to four chemicals in chanca piedra: niranthin, nirtetralin, hinokinin, and geraniin.

In subsequent research, strong antiviral actions have been reported for other unique *Phyllanthus* compounds called phyllanthin and hypophyllanthin. With all the confusion of disparate studies, the Cochrane Hepato-Biliary Research Group in Copenhagen reviewed all the published HBV research in 2001 (22 randomized trials) and published an independent review of the results. It stated that treatment with "*Phyllanthus* herb" (they acknowledged the confusion among the various species used) had "a positive effect on clearance of serum HBsAg" (HBV surface antigen) comparable to interferon and was better than nonspecific treatment or other herbal medicines for HBV and liver enzyme normalization."

In addition to the confusion about the different results based on which *Phyllanthus* herb was used, there was great variety in how the plants were processed or extracted, which, in turn, had an enormous influence on the antiviral abilities demonstrated in various studies. This trend has continued over the last 20 years with the development of many more extraction processes using some type of alcohol. Because chanca piedra cannot be patented as a proprietary product that would justify the high cost of funding research, many different water or alcohol extracts have been created and studied, which are now being sold around the world as herbal drugs. Each manufacturer is using its own proprietary extraction process to extract the herb; many of these products or extraction methods are patented now. Unfortunately, when you delve into the antiviral studies, many of these proprietary products just don't work as well as the natural plant did when it was first confirmed with antiviral actions against hepatitis as a simple herbal tea. When I sorted through the many studies, this is what I found: When whole-herb chanca piedra is administered as a tea or provided in capsules or extracted in water, it has the highest antiviral effect. Nevertheless, proprietary and patented herbal drugs of chanca piedra or (*Phyllanthus amarus*) now exist in Italy, Germany, India, Malaysia and Indonesia with most being marketed for the treatment of hepatitis as well as kidney stones.

These products have been the subject of research in the last several years, including for their antiviral actions. Researchers in Malaysia published a study in 2019 reporting that an alcohol extract of chanca piedra was effective *in vitro* against hepatitis C. Researchers in India reported the same antiviral ability *in vitro* and in mice with *Phyllanthus amarus* inhibiting hepatitis C in 2017 and *in vitro* in 2011. In the 2017 research, they extracted a compound called corilagin from the plant (also found in higher amounts in chanca piedra) and tested it individually, reporting that it had very strong anti–hepatitis C actions in very low dosages. A university research group in Italy conducted a randomized, controlled human trial on the patented Italian chanca piedra herbal drug for hepatitis B infection in 2018. They reported that no significant differences in viral load were found between the herbal drug intervention and placebo groups after 12 months and 24 months, and no subjects showed HBsAg clearance.

Chanca piedra has also shown antiviral actions against other viruses. Concerned with HIV specifically, a Japanese research group reported that a simple water extract of chanca piedra inhibited HIV-1 reverse transcriptase in

1992. (Several conventional drugs used today against HIV are classified as "reverse transcriptase inhibitors.") They attributed this effect to a plant chemical in chanca piedra called repandusinic acid A. When they tested this chemical individually, it demonstrated significant toxicity to HIV-1 at very small dosages (a 90 percent *in vitro* inhibition using only 2.5 micrograms). Bristol Myers Squibb Pharmaceutical Research Institute isolated yet another chemical in chanca piedra with anti-HIV actions—a novel compound that they named niruriside and described in a 1996 study. A German research organization published their first study on chanca piedra and its application with HIV therapy (reporting a 70 to 75 percent inhibition of virus) in 2003.

In addition, several studies published between 2007 and 2011 report that chanca piedra can inhibit the growth of various herpes viruses. Newer research reports that chanca piedra may be beneficial for treating a tropical viral infection carried by mosquitos called *dengue virus* which causes dengue fever.

My personal experience using chanca piedra for viruses evolved over many years. I believe that chanca piedra is an important therapy for hepatitis because the virus is causing significant damage to the liver. Chanca piedra is one of the best herbal remedies for the liver—to prevent damage, heal damaged liver cells, and promote the regenerative ability of the liver to produce new healthy liver cells. More about chanca piedra's benefits to the liver will be discussed in the next chapter. I've used chanca piedra as a monotherapy for hepatitis B with some good results but most often combined it with other antiviral plants for clients with hepatitis C. As rainforest shamans have taught me, combining several plants together usually results in better actions. I developed an herbal antiviral formula called Amazon A-V years ago that contained chanca piedra along with other effective Amazon antiviral plants, which I used much more often for all viruses than chanca piedra alone.

I've always believed the synergistic action of multiple natural compounds working together are more effective than just a few, especially when dealing with tricky microbes that can mutate to be resistant to compounds trying to kill them. However, for the hepatitis viruses, my protocol usually added extra chanca piedra (2 grams daily) to the A-V multi-herb formula, which provided excellent results for both hepatitis B and C, including active and recent infections, as well as long-standing chronic infections. Helping to protect and heal the liver with extra chanca piedra was thought to immediately address liver issues during initial or chronic infections, and it could help clear the liver more effectively from dead and dying viral cells with chanca piedra's liver-detoxing actions.

Many integrative and alternative health practitioners relied on the multi-herb formula to treat their patients in a similar fashion with good results. The formula also worked very well for herpes viruses. While it was able to reduce viral loads of HIV by up to 80 percent, it wasn't able to clear the virus completely. More information on the Amazon A-V formula and how to prepare it is in the resource section.

Chanca piedra is one of the better herbal antivirals available as an herbal remedy. Its ability to interfere with protease will negatively affect most all types of viruses because, without adequate protease, viruses cannot divide and multiply rapidly. That chanca piedra also stimulates the immune system to seek out and destroy these invading viruses more quickly and efficiently is just more good news for those faced with a viral infection.

Chanca Piedra and Evolving Flu Viruses

One of the main emerging pathogens that affects everyone are new evolving viruses we are faced with. The latest of these is the COVID-19 coronavirus that originated in China in the winter of 2019 and by early 2020 had spread to the rest of the world and classified as a pandemic virus. Other similar pandemic viruses had come before such as swine flu (H1N2), bird flu (H5N1), SARS, and MERS. There have been many different types of coronavirus flu outbreaks, with the first recorded in 1965. SARS (severe acute respiratory syndrome) emerged in 2002 to 2003 as a coronavirus from southern China and spread throughout the world with quantifiable speed much like COVID-19 did. Coronaviruses can infect humans and animals equally, and many of the new pathogenic strains of these pandemic viruses usually begin with transmission from animal to human, and all can mutate quickly once they reside in humans.

Personally, every time a new flu virus breaks out, I make sure I have plenty of chanca piedra on hand. Various *in vitro* tests confirm chanca piedra is an effective antiviral against various strains of flu virus, and I've used it successfully against previous swine and bird flu strains. This newest COVID-19 viral strain is a bit different from those that came before it, and its difference makes chanca piedra even more important. This new strain of flu immediately attacks the lungs, and poor outcomes usually result from what is called a "cytokine storm" reaction in people, which causes significant damage to the lungs, as I mentioned in the introduction to this book. Cytokines are the types of pro-inflammatory immune cells discussed earlier in chanca piedra's immunomodulatory actions. When a virus overstimulates an immune reaction, the inflammation the cytokines causes can result in cell damage to the lungs on top of the cell death the actual virus causes in the lungs. As discussed earlier, chanca piedra can modulate these immune responses, lowering production of these inflammatory cytokines, while increasing other non-inflammatory cells responsible for killing the virus. This makes chanca piedra a very good natural remedy to try for this particular viral strain.

Chanca piedra has not been scientifically tested to be capable of directly killing this particular coronavirus like it can others, but it's immunomodulatory actions alone had me stocking up on chanca piedra, just in case. You'll also learn in the next chapter how chanca piedra's cellular-protective antioxidant actions play a beneficial role in helping to protect cells and organs from cellular damage. The protective action of chanca piedra to the lungs has already been established in human studies studying chanca piedra in people with pneumonia and tuberculosis. This new flu virus damages the lungs, and the resulting inflammation can promote the development of pneumonia, which usually results in the need for hospitalization, breathing assistance, and increased mortality rates over other viral strains. That chanca piedra might interrupt this process, was again, enough for me to stock up on chanca piedra during this recent pandemic with COVID-19.

While every year the drug companies create flu vaccines, their effectiveness is usually less than 50 percent. They just can't determine which flu strains might surface in any given year, and the viruses mutate so quickly and regularly, it's simply a guessing game as to which particular strain of virus should be included in a vaccine. I'll always have chanca piedra on hand when flu season arrives for that reason.

Antibacterial, Antifungal, and Antiparasitic Actions

In addition to killing viruses effectively, research reports that chanca piedra can kill disease-causing bacteria, yeast (*Candida*), and several parasites. The plant's ability to treat candida yeast infections in women were confirmed through a randomized, double-blind, controlled study published in 2006. The research group who performed the study in India were also inspired by the plant's reported immunomodulation abilities and recorded the immune responses in 30 women with candida infections treated with chanca piedra. They reported that chanca piedra worked slightly better at curing the yeast infection than a drug they used as a control and also reported immune function and, specifically, immunity was much enhanced in those taking chanca piedra. There was a significantly lower rate of reoccurring candida infections noted in the women receiving chanca piedra, even after three months of the initial treatment. Even though further larger clinical studies are needed, the result of this preliminary study with chanca piedra was in line with the approach of other research that reports that immunotherapy is beneficial in patients with reoccurring vaginal yeast infections in both speeding up the recovery as well preventing chronic reoccurrence.

More than 28 studies published between 1983 and

2020 report that chanca piedra (and *Phyllanthus amarus*) has strong antibacterial actions. These studies are preliminary *in vitro* studies that introduce the plants to various disease-causing bacteria in a test tube to determine which bacteria it can kill directly. This doesn't always relate to how the herb might kill bacteria in human or animals; therefore, it's simply a starting point for researchers to design animal studies to re-create the *in vitro* results. Only two animal studies have been conducted thus far and are discussed next.

The *in vitro* research indicates if chanca piedra comes in direct contact with bacteria, it kills a large variety of gram-positive and gram-negative bacteria (including multi-drug-resistant strains), mycobacteria and mycoplasmas, and even spirochete-type bacteria. Lyme disease and syphilis are a type of spirochete bacteria, and tuberculosis and pneumonia are representative of mycobacteria and mycoplasma, respectively. Both water and alcohol extracts of the plants had antibacterial actions, and for once, the alcohol extracts were reported with slightly stronger actions than water extracts. Chanca piedra had slightly better results against bacteria than *Phyllanthus amarus* did, and both killed a much larger variety of gram-positive bacteria than gram-negative strains.

Interestingly, the probiotic friendly strains of bacteria (*Lactobacillus* and *bacillus*) were not affected by chanca piedra's antibiotic actions. The common food contaminate strains of bacteria, *Salmonella, E. coli,* and *Listeria,* were all susceptible to the herb's antibacterial actions, which some scientists reported may be indicative of the herb's potential to be a natural antimicrobial food preservative. Three bacterial strains in the human mouth linked to the development of cavities were also killed by chanca piedra. Several types of natural compounds are attributed to the plant's ability to kill bacteria, including polyphenols, alkaloids, and saponins with over a dozen antimicrobial plant compounds identified in the plant thus far.

One animal study conducted in 2020 in the West African country of Benin studied the ability of *Phyllanthus amarus* to treat salmonella infections in baby chickens. They reported that a water extract reduced the bacterial load of chicks with lab-induced salmonella infection by 52.38 percent. Researchers in Indonesia studied chanca piedra given to chickens with a mycoplasma infection in 2018. They reported effective antibacterial effects as well as lowered inflammation and higher immune cell activation similar to the studies conducted on chanca piedra's immunomodulatory studies.

Chanca piedra (and *Phyllanthus amarus*) have also shown in research to have antimalarial and antiparasitic actions against several common tropical diseases. Malaria is caused by a *Plasmodium* parasite that is transmitted through mosquitos. Schistosomiasis is caused by a tropical blood fluke parasite, *Schistosoma mansoni,* transmitted through snails. Leishmaniasis is a tropical disease caused by a *Leishmania* parasite transmitted through sandflies. These two *Phyllanthus* plants are the subject of 25 studies over the last 20 years that report the plants provide antiparasitic actions against all three of these common parasites. The *in vitro* studies report strong actions; however, the animal studies conducted thus far indicate that chanca piedra can reduce parasitic burden by around 50 to 70 percent, depending on the parasite. These parasites go through several growth stages during their life span, and chanca piedra plants aren't as effective in some of the later stages.

CHAPTER 5

Chanca Piedra's Many Other Benefits

In addition to the benefits discussed in the previous chapters, chanca piedra has many effective traditional uses for a wide variety of diseases. Some of the traditional medicinal usages have been proven in experimental models, which confirm that this herbal remedy possesses various pharmacological actions. Some of these benefits and uses have been evaluated in human trials for the treatment of hypertension, jaundice, diabetes, and viral infections. This chapter will provide an overview of the research conducted on chanca piedra, which helps form the basis for the natural remedy protocols for this impressive South American herbal remedy.

Antioxidant Actions

Chanca piedra has been the subject of a great deal of recent research on the plant's antioxidant actions. In more than 20 different studies, chanca piedra evidenced strong antioxidant actions. As discussed earlier, natural polyphenol compounds are very effective antioxidants, and chanca piedra contains more than 70 polyphenols with even more metabolites being formed during digestion when the herb is consumed. Polyphenol amounts can vary in plants based on growing conditions and time of harvest, as well as on how scientist extract the plants to measure the amount of polyphenols the sample contains. Tests on chanca piedra report that total polyphenols in the plant range from 164 to 224 milligrams of polyphenols in 1 gram of dried chanca piedra.

That chanca piedra has antioxidant actions is pretty much a given in light of the number and amount of natural polyphenol chemicals it provides. Other non-polyphenol plant compounds in chanca piedra also contribute its antioxidant action. Some of these compounds lend electrons to free radicals to convert them to stable molecules, which stops their damaging actions. Others are effective enzyme-inhibitors and can interfere and disable the enzymes that are needed to actually create a new free radical, thereby reducing the amount of free radicals in our bodies. Standard antioxidants tests have been conducted on chanca piedra confirming its strong antioxidant abilities.

In 2014 Brazilian researchers gave five healthy nonsmokers a chanca piedra tea to determine what it effect it had on their antioxidant markers in their bloodstream. Plasma levels of gallic acid were significantly increased at one, two, and four hours of taking the tea, and plasma ascorbic acid was higher at one hour after ingestion. Gallic acid is one of the main polyphenolic acids in chanca piedra and is a well-known antioxidant capable of disabling free radicals in human and animals. Vitamin C is the most studied of all vitamin antioxidants our bodies need for a healthy antioxidant system as well as a healthy immune system.

These researchers summarized their research saying that the increase in these antioxidant markers in human blood may contribute to chanca piedra's pharmacological effects.

Another study was conducted in 2015 on *Phyllanthus amarus*. This plant variety has fewer polyphenols than chanca piedra does. Exercise is known to temporarily increase free radicals since exercise increases respiration. As free radicals are a byproduct of turning the oxygen we breathe into the type cellular oxygen our cells can use, free radicals increase as respiration increases. For that reason, many antioxidant studies in humans use exercise models. Researchers in Thailand measured the antioxidant status of 12 healthy but sedentary men participating in single session of moderate-intensity exercise through cycling. They reported that their study confirmed the beneficial effect of *Phyllanthus amarus* supplementation, which improves antioxidant status. They also reported much higher plasma levels of vitamin C immediately after high-intensity exercise, which resulted in decreased fat oxidation (lipid peroxidation) and muscle soreness two days later.

See the reference section for a listing of the published studies on chanca piedra's antioxidant actions.

Cellular-Protective Antioxidant Actions

In addition to interfering in the production of free radicals and lending electrons to turn free radicals into stable molecules, chanca piedra has shown the ability to protect cells and organs from oxidative stress, relieve inflammation, and even repair cells that have been damaged by free radicals and/or chronic inflammation. Research reveals that chanca piedra provided cellular-protective antioxidant actions, which protect various cells and organs from known oxidative damage by various drugs, toxins, and free radicals. These studies show that chanca piedra can protect brain cells, kidneys, liver, stomach lining, heart, intestines, and muscles from oxidative stress, cellular damage, and resulting inflammation.

The research on chanca piedra's kidney-protective action and its ability to relieve oxidative stress and protect the kidneys from known toxins was discussed in chapter 3. A significant amount of research (more than 70 studies) has been conducted in animals and humans confirming chanca piedra's ability to relieve oxidative stress, as well as protect and repair the liver from oxidative damage and introduced toxins. This research is discussed later in this chapter under "Liver-Protective Actions."

Researchers often use diabetic animal models to determine if a plant or a drug has cellular-protective antioxidant actions. Diabetes not only causes significant increases in blood sugar, triglycerides, total cholesterol, creatinine, and urea levels but also provokes high oxidative stress in the pancreas and kidneys, which can be easily measured. Three studies have been conducted that report that chanca piedra can effectively protect rodents from the oxidative stress diabetes causes to the pancreas and kidneys. The latest study was published in 2020 by Indian researchers, and they attributed these results to chanca piedra's antioxidant and anti-inflammatory polyphenols.

Several other studies report that chanca piedra can protect the stomach and digestive tract from various introduced chemicals and toxins that damage and/or ulcerate the stomach lining. Other researchers induced oxidative stress and inflammation in the brains of mice and rats and reported that chanca piedra could protect brain cells from damage, reduce brain cell death, and lower oxidative stress and inflammation in the brains of the animals. Additionally, several chemotherapy drugs used in cancer treatment cause toxicity, cellular damage, and oxidative stress to the heart or renal system. Several studies suggest chanca piedra could be used in combination with these drugs as their animal research suggested the plant could protect these organs from the normal damage these drugs cause. Chanca piedra has also been reported to be effective in protecting various cells from radiation damage as well.

While most researchers attribute these cellular-protective actions to the plant's many protective polyphenols, a research group in India reported in 2014 that chanca piedra's proteins (made up by amino acids) were effective antioxidant and anti-inflammatory substances that protected rodents from liver damage and oxidative stress caused by high doses of aspirin in their research.

Whatever natural compounds are involved, it's obvious from the research that chanca piedra provides excellent cellular-protective actions that could be beneficial in numerous health conditions, including remediating the negative effects of various pharmaceutical drugs used to treat these conditions.

Anti-Inflammatory & Pain-Relieving Actions

Another well-studied action of chanca piedra is the plant's ability to relieve pain. This action was well noted in the human studies with patients with kidney stones and gout who reported pain relief, and 18 other studies published between 1994 and 2019 have confirmed chanca piedra's pain-relieving actions. Various models of induced pain in laboratory animals report that chanca piedra relieved chronic and acute pain, nerve and muscle pain, and sciatica and neuropathic pain, as well as topical and internal pain. One study with mice reported that a water extract of chanca piedra was equal to that of the common pain drug tramadol. Another study with mice reported that chanca piedra was effective at relieving the pain of diabetic neuropathy. Thus far, at least nine different active chemical compounds have been individually tested with pain-relieving actions, and it is most likely that these chemicals are working together synergistically to provide this pain-relief action.

Some of this research studying pain additionally studied chanca piedra's anti-inflammatory actions and other research focused solely on inflammation. A total of 16 animal studies and two human studies confirm that chanca piedra has effective anti-inflammatory benefits. The plant is reported to relieve inflammation in several different ways, including modulating and downregulating various pro-inflammatory immune responses and chemicals, relieving oxidative stress (which causes inflammation), and reducing the production of various other inflammatory chemicals and processes through four different pathways. Two studies reported that chanca piedra's antibacterial action against several strains of bacteria, which produce a chemical called lipopolysaccharide (LPS), was effective in relieving the inflammation typically caused by LPS. Various models of laboratory-induced inflammation to muscles, joints, brain, stomach, throat, and liver were studied, and it was reported in these studies that chanca piedra offers broad-spectrum anti-inflammatory benefits in all models studied.

As discussed in the previous chapter; if you reduce free radicals and the cellular damage and oxidative stress they cause, the levels of chronic inflammation is reduced. It's obvious from the anti-inflammatory research that this type of inflammation relief is achieved; however, chanca piedra employs other mechanisms for inflammation relief as well. One of these mechanisms is by modulating the immune response discussed previously.

Liver-Protective Actions

The benefits of chanca piedra for the liver is another subject that has been established with clinical research in animals and humans. A huge amount of recent research has been conducted on chanca piedra's ability to benefit the liver, protect it from various drugs, toxins, and diseases, and reduce or eliminate the risks of developing fatty liver and liver cancer. These effects have been attributed to herb's many protective polyphenols as well as to two novel plant chemicals in chanca piedra, phyllanthin and hypophyllanthin, and another natural compound, corilagin. More than 70 research studies have now confirmed chanca piedra's benefits to detoxify, protect, and heal the liver.

When scientists began testing individual compounds in chanca piedra in 2019, they determined that quite a few compounds protected the liver, and those producing the highest liver-protective benefits were the compounds corilagin, isocorilagin, kaempferol rhamnoside, and brevifolin carboxylic acid. However, chanca piedra's overall strong cellular-protective antioxidant action, which is delivered though many compounds working together synergistically, is one of the main mechanisms of actions the herb uses to help protect and heal the liver. Almost all the published research on chanca piedra's liver-protective abilities speak of the herb's ability to reduce oxidative stress, cellular damage, and inflammation in the liver.

The liver is a vital organ that controls many aspects of health. The liver controls most chemical levels in the bloodstream. It also secretes bile, which helps to break down fats, preparing them for further digestion and absorption. All the blood leaving the stomach and intestines passes through the liver. The liver processes this blood and breaks down, balances, and creates nutrients for the body to use. It also breaks down (metabolizes) medicines in the blood into forms that are easier for the body to use. When the liver has broken down harmful substances, they are excreted into the bile or blood. Bile byproducts enter the intestine and ultimately leave the body in bowel movements. Blood byproducts are filtered out by the kidneys and leave the body in the form of urine.

The liver carries out many important functions: it produces bile, which helps carry away waste and break down fats in the small intestine during digestion; makes certain proteins for blood plasma; makes cholesterol and special proteins to help carry fats through the body; stores and releases glucose as needed; changes harmful ammonia to urea (a byproduct of protein metabolism that is excreted in the urine); clears the blood of medicines, chemical toxins, and other harmful substances; regulates blood clotting; and fights infections by making immune factors and removing bacteria from the bloodstream.

To measure the function and health of the liver, several blood tests are performed as part of a standard liver function panel. Liver dysfunction can elevate or change any of the following parameters:

- ❑ **Alanine aminotransferase (ALT):** Elevated ALT helps identify liver disease or damage from any number of causes.
- ❑ **Aspartate aminotransferase (AST):** Elevated AST checks for liver damage.
- ❑ **Alkaline phosphatase:** Alkaline phosphatase is present in bile-secreting cells in the liver; it's also in bones. High levels often mean bile flow out of the liver is blocked or reduced.
- ❑ **Bilirubin:** High bilirubin levels suggest a problem with the liver.
- ❑ **Albumin:** As part of total protein levels, albumin helps determine how well the liver is working.
- ❑ **Ammonia:** Ammonia levels in the blood rise when the liver is not functioning properly.

When the liver is damaged by free radicals, it can also suffer from chronic inflammation. Free radicals are circulating in the bloodstream, and the blood is filtered by the liver, exposing the liver to the damage free radicals cause. Free radicals are also a byproduct of digestion; they move into the bloodstream from the intestines and go directly to the liver for filtration. Therefore, the liver is highly susceptible to free radical damage. This damage and resulting low level of chronic inflammation can affect the liver's ability to do its job efficiently.

For example, when the liver isn't functioning properly due to excess free radical damage and chronic inflammation, it cannot efficiently process fats. As a result, fat accumulates in the liver and causes hepatic stenosis, or fatty liver. The significant elevation in free radical levels and the damage they cause in obesity, type 2 diabetes, and excessive alcohol consumption often overwhelms our built-in antioxidant system along with the natural antioxidants our bodies produce to keep free radicals at healthy levels. Free radicals circulating in the blood cause oxidative stress to the liver, and all three of these high free radical conditions are well known to cause fatty liver. In addition, a chronically inflamed liver can also raise cholesterol levels and produce too many triglycerides, and because free radicals are present in the liver, it becomes a significant site in the body where a large amount of cholesterol is oxidized, which is linked to the development of clogged arteries.

Additionally, hepatitis is actually defined as inflammation of the liver. However, this sort of inflammation is more pronounced than the lower level of chronic inflammation that free radicals cause. Viruses cause most cases of hepatitis and are named by which virus is infecting the liver: hepatitis A, B, or C. The inflammation in the liver caused by these viruses results in liver malfunction, which leads to liver damage, and sometimes this damage leads to the development of liver cancer. In any regard, the blood parameters in the liver panel test are all elevated in hepatitis patients (and animals), which is the main method doctors use to determine how much liver damage the virus is causing.

When researchers go into their laboratories to test the liver-protective or repairing ability of chanca piedra and other natural plants and compounds, they employ the standard liver panel of blood tests. Typically, they run a baseline test to confirm the liver blood levels are normal; they damage the liver with various chemicals and/or toxins and run another liver panel test to confirm damage caused by the substance they gave the animals. They then treat the animals with chanca piedra for a period of time and run the blood test again to compare how these liver levels were affected, which relates to the reduction of damage provided by the plant. These tests indicate that a substance like chanca piedra has a healing and repairing action.

Alternatively, there are well-known chemicals with known liver-damaging effects that researchers will give animals in combination with chanca piedra to determine if the plant could prevent the damage that normally occurs. This type of research usually has two groups of animals: one that receives the plant with the toxin and a control group that receives just the toxin. In some studies, researchers pretreated one group of animals with chanca piedra, administered the drug or toxin, and then measured the amount of protection provided by chanca piedra compared to a control group. Researchers then compared the liver damage based on the liver panel test between the two groups of animals. This type of research indicates that chanca piedra has a protective effect on the liver.

The last type of test researchers use to determine liver-protective abilities utilizes diabetic animals. Diabetes significantly raises free radical levels; the resulting cellular damage and chronic inflammation negatively affects liver function (measured by liver panel test results). In these studies, scientists induce diabetes in the animals using a pancreatic-damaging chemical and then measure the oxidative stress in the liver and resulting damage in a control group compared to another group of animals receiving chanca piedra. This method also confirms the plant's ability to prevent the normal damage to the liver that diabetes usually causes. Some researchers even used chanca piedra to treat the liver damage in diabetic animals after the diabetes caused liver damage for a longer period of time.

More than 40 animal studies have been conducted on chanca piedra using these test models to validate the plant's liver-protecting and liver-healing actions. The liver toxins used in the research included various chemotherapy drugs, environmental toxins, high levels of alcohol and aspirin, and other standard chemicals or drugs known to cause liver damage. Many of these studies reported 100 percent protection depending on the toxin administered and others reported significant protection (up to 80 percent). Other research confirmed chanca piedra's ability to repair the damage these chemicals caused. Again, in most studies, researchers reported significant improvements and even normalization of blood parameters measured with the standard liver panel tests after chanca piedra was administered to animals with damaged livers. Several studies reported that chanca piedra completely protected animals from developing fatty liver disease, and some reported that it treated it effectively after it was induced in animals.

Some researchers in this body of liver research monitored

oxidation and antioxidant levels in animals, and reported a significant reduction of free radicals and restoration of natural enzyme antioxidant levels that are usually reduced when the body is fighting free radicals naturally and becomes reduced due to the high level of circulating free radicals. Other researchers monitored inflammation levels in the liver and/or pro-inflammatory chemicals circulating in the bloodstream and reported that chanca piedra significantly reduced inflammation (chronic and acute) and lowered pro-inflammatory immune chemicals as described and previously discussed in chanca piedra's immunomodulatory actions.

A handful of studies looked at the negative effect alcohol has on the liver, which promotes the development of cirrhosis. The research reported that in the presence of high alcohol, chanca piedra prevented cirrhosis in animals, and when administered to animals with liver cirrhosis, it significantly improved the condition and encouraged the development of new liver cells to replace those that were damaged.

The liver is unique among all organs because it is programmed to regenerate quickly and liver cells in general are short lived and are being constantly replaced. Unlike any other organs, someone can donate a portion of their liver (up to one-third) to someone needing a liver transplant, and their liver will quickly regenerate and replace the portion that was removed within just a couple of months. Researchers have reported that chanca piedra encourages and promotes this regeneration process, and speeds the development of new liver cells, which can be helpful to replace damaged liver cells more quickly in numerous types of liver disorders. Recent *in vitro* research in 2019 reports that chanca piedra and three of its active compounds (phyllanthin, hypophyllanthin, and gallic acid) interferes with and inhibits the enzyme in the liver that breaks down alcohol for absorption.

The overwhelming evidence in the animal research indicates that chanca piedra is a highly effective natural remedy for the liver, and like most of the other research, the use of water extracts or just feeding animals the herb or a herbal tea produced better results than alcohol extracts or some of the other proprietary extracts developed that used alcohol. A study published in 2019 compared the liver-protective actions of various extracts of chanca piedra. They noted the strongest actions in the water extracts, and it was important to note that the 50, 70 and 80 percent ethanol extracts offered no protection against the chemical toxin they studied (Carbon tetrachloride or CCl4).

These liver-protective and healing effects have also been confirmed in human studies. Most all of the 30-some-odd human studies for hepatitis monitored liver function and injury of study subjects through the standard liver panel of blood tests. Almost without exception, chanca piedra had a beneficial effect on improving the numbers in these tests. Even when a particular chanca piedra extract or proprietary extract they used failed to significantly lower the hepatitis viral load, it often still provided some sort of liver protection benefits and/or increased liver function. For that reason, even when conflicting research suggested that an extract used wasn't treating the viral infection, it was still treating the liver inflammation and function, so more research continued to be funded and conducted. Several of the early hepatitis human studies using just chanca piedra tea reported all liver injury markers in this standard blood test returned to normal levels.

Two human studies reported chanca piedra's liver-protective and detoxifying actions in children with hepatitis and jaundice. Indian researchers reported that chanca piedra was an effective single drug in the treatment of jaundice in children, and British researchers reported that children treated with a chanca piedra extract for acute hepatitis had liver function return to normal within five days. Researchers in China also reported liver-protective actions when chanca piedra was given to adults with chronic hepatitis.

Interestingly, a proprietary water and alcohol extract of *Phyllanthus amarus* is sold in Malaysia and was the subject of a small randomized, double-blind, placebo-controlled crossover study in 2019. Fifteen healthy subjects were recruited and half were given the *Phyllanthus* product for 10 days and then all subjects drank enough alcohol to create a hangover. They measured levels of oxidative stress, liver damage, and hangover symptoms between both groups. The results indicated the product was able to remove blood alcohol in the pretreated group while the control group still had 0.05 percent at 12 hours post-intoxication. It was also shown to lower oxidative stress and inflammation levels and to reduce the number and severity of hangover symptoms over the control group.

My personal experience using chanca piedra for liver disorders indicated it really did provide great benefits for the liver. I used it often for liver protection and detoxification. However, I developed a liver-specific multi-herb remedy with chanca piedra as the main ingredient, Amazon Liver Support, for more severe liver disorders. It was well regarded and used by many practitioners. I always recall one rather dramatic occasion when I talk about the liver support formula. A client who had liver failure as a result of a clinical trial he had participated in was referred to me by another practitioner. The clinical trial combined two antiviral drugs, which both had liver toxicity, for the treatment of AIDS. It was conducted in Austin, Texas, where my company and I were located at the time. The trial was suspended prior to completion as the patients experienced significant liver damage, and most ended up on the Texas liver transplant waiting list.

I gave the client the Amazon Liver Support formula along with extra chanca piedra. This was often my protocol when I needed significant liver regeneration quickly. The client had immediate improvement and referred two other people from the clinical trial. All three were removed from the transplant list and recovered completely in fewer than 60 days. It was truly remarkable, which is why it is so memorable.

The liver formula also had a large following for liver cirrhosis. An Austin chapter coordinator for Alcoholics Anonymous was referred to me in 2004 by their practitioner. He had significant improvements in his liver cirrhosis and normalized his liver enzyme levels with the formula. He spread the word far and wide within the AA organization about his positive results, which kept demand strong for this particular effective formula for cirrhosis of the liver. More information about the Amazon Liver Support formula, required dosages, and how to make it is found in the resource section.

The naturopathic protocol for chanca piedra for overall liver support and prevention is 2 grams daily in capsules or prepared as a tea. For liver protection and healing during hepatitis, cirrhosis, diabetes, other diseases that elevate liver enzymes, or in combination with necessary liver-toxic drugs, take three 500-milligram capsules three times daily. If you weigh more than 185 pounds, take four 500-milligram capsules three times daily. If desired, two cups of a standard chanca piedra tea (with 1 teaspoon herb powder per cup) daily can be substituted. See the consumer guide in the next chapter concerning contraindications, drug interactions, and other important information if you are currently using prescription drugs.

Cancer Prevention & Anticancer Actions

Chanca piedra's cancer preventative and anticancer actions have been documented in 15 test-tube studies and several animal studies. All the anticancer research is preliminary, and most are *in vitro* studies—introducing chanca piedra to various cancer cells in test tubes to determine which types of cancer cells are killed and how. This preliminary research reveals that the types of cancer cells most susceptible to the actions of the chanca piedra in these studies include leukemia, colorectal, liver, cervical, prostate, and ovarian cancer cells Some of this research reported that chanca piedra could kill these cancer cells in dosages as small as 8 micrograms (0.08 milligrams). This research also reports that chanca piedra selectively kills the cancer cells in a dose-dependent manner without damage or cell death to healthy cells. In several *in vitro* research studies, chanca piedra has also been shown to have antimetastatic and antiproliferative actions against breast, lung, melanoma, and osteosarcoma cancer cells. It didn't kill these types of cancer outright; rather, it inhibited the growth and/or spread.

Much more research is required to demonstrate if chanca piedra is capable of treating cancer. This type of research usually begins with animal studies to try to verify and confirm the research performed *in vitro*. If animal studies are successful, only then will human studies be considered. Only a handful of animal studies have been conducted on chanca piedra's anticancer and or cancer-preventative actions thus far.

A 2000 study documented that chanca piedra increased the life span of mice with liver cancer from 33 weeks (control group without treatment) to 52 weeks. Another research group tried to induce liver cancer in mice that had been pretreated with a water extract of chanca piedra. Their results indicated the chanca piedra extract dose-dependently lowered tumor incidence, levels of carcinogen-metabolizing enzymes, levels of liver cancer markers, and levels of liver injury markers. Other *in vitro* and animal studies suggest that chanca piedra can reduce the risk of developing liver cancer.

Researchers in India reported in 2009 and again in 2011 that chanca piedra protected mice from skin cancer when they gave animals oral dosages of chanca piedra before, during, or after inducing skin cancer in the animals. Tumor incidence was greatly reduced in all three administration periods. Their 2011 study reported that chanca piedra's strong antioxidant actions were measured and verified, and the cancer-prevention abilities with regard to skin cancers were probably due to chanca piedra's strong antioxidant abilities to prevent the cellular damage that would result in the mutation of skin cells into cancerous cells.

New research on cancer has reported a causal and functional connection between inflammation and certain types of cancer, and it has become a subject of much research interest. Researchers are looking for compounds able to modulate inflammation-related signaling pathways in anticancer drug development programs as a new way to treat cancer. Chanca piedra has surfaced in this new search as a possible candidate. A group of researchers from the United States, Malaysia, and India published a study in 2020 that reported: "Plants possessing anticancer and anti-inflammatory properties due to their bioactive constituents have been reported to modulate the molecular and cellular pathways which are related to inflammation and cancer. In this review we focus on the flavonoids (astragalin, kaempferol, quercetin, rutin), lignans (phyllanthin, hypophyllanthin, and niranthin), tannins (corilagin, geraniin, ellagic acid, gallic acid), and triterpenes (lupeol, oleanolic acid, ursolic acid) of *Phyllanthus amarus*, which exert various anticancer and anti-inflammatory activities via perturbation of the NF-κB, MAPKs, PI3K/Akt, and Wnt signaling networks."

The tannin polyphenol in chanca piedra called corilagin has been the subject of recent cancer research and some researchers believe the high amount of corilagin in chanca piedra (which is higher in chanca piedra than in *Phyllanthus amarus*) is responsible for much of the antitumor actions demonstrated in test-tube research on the plant. However, other *Phyllanthus* compounds called phyllanthin and geraniin have also been studied individually for their effective anticancer actions *in vitro* as well. As with most all research on plants, once scientists determine which natural compounds provide the highest anticancer effects, future research dollars are spent on these chemical compounds rather than on the plant itself. These compounds can result in new patented cancer drugs unlike the natural plant, which cannot be patented.

Several *in vitro* studies as well as the animal studies report that chanca piedra might provide cancer-preventative actions due to its antimutagenic actions. When healthy cells are exposed to various cancer-causing toxic chemicals and/or exposed to free radical damage, it can cause DNA damage to the cell, which promotes the cell to mutate into a cancer cell. Several test-tube studies report that chanca piedra prevented healthy cells from mutating into cancerous cells when given a substance known to create mutations. The animal studies reported cancer-prevention abilities along the same lines for skin cancer and liver cancer as well. Many of the strong cellular-protective antioxidant polyphenols in chanca piedra have been shown to have good antimutagenic actions in other studies, so is not surprising that chanca piedra evidenced this cancer-preventative action. Tens of thousands of studies over the last 20 years confirm the general cancer-prevention abilities of plant antioxidants, including several polyphenols and flavonoids found in chanca piedra.

After poring through all the new cancer research on chanca piedra, my original opinions formed before this new research was conducted hasn't changed very much. I never used or recommended chanca piedra as a stand-alone remedy to treat cancer. Based on the research I'm reading today, it might slow cancer growth and maybe reduce or prevent some cancers from metastasizing or spreading, and its real benefits are for the possible prevention of cancer through several mechanisms of action. I did, however, often use chanca piedra or one of the chanca piedra multi-herb formulas as an adjunctive supplement for liver cancer and urinary tract cancers in combination with a multi-herb formula I created with Amazon plants with anticancer actions called N-Tense. I knew chanca piedra was having a beneficial effect on the liver and kidneys, and was capable of treating oxidative stress in both organs, which is significantly elevated in cancer. However, I was mainly relying on the anticancer actions of the multi-herb anticancer formula and not chanca piedra specifically. I must note, however, liver cancer was one of the most remarkable results I've seen in all my years of helping cancer patients. The combination of the chanca piedra–rich liver support formula (Amazon Liver Support) in combination with the N-Tense formula created more remissions and cures than seen in any other type of cancer.

Anti-Aging and AGE-Inhibitor Actions

As discussed in previous chapters, aging has been associated with a chronic low-grade inflammatory state as well as increased oxidative stress. It is widely accepted that reactive oxygen species (ROS) in many cells accumulate over our life span and lead to a state of chronic oxidative stress at old age. Low-grade inflammation caused by oxidative stress is also now strongly linked to much higher risks of developing age-related memory loss, dementia, and even Alzheimer's disease. Chanca piedra's strong antioxidant actions to fight free radicals, including ROS, and relieve oxidative stress and chronic inflammation are at the core of chanca piedra's ability to promote healthy aging.

However, another huge area of anti-aging research over the last 10 years indicates that reducing advanced glycation end products (AGEs) in the body provides anti-aging benefits. AGEs are harmful compounds that are formed when protein or fat combines or bonds improperly with sugar in the bloodstream. This process is called glycation. These improperly bonded compounds can travel throughout the body and cause a host of problems, including chronic inflammation, cellular damage and cell death, and the interruption of cellular signaling. AGEs also encourage the creation of ROS, which generate oxidative stress and more inflammation. In fact, AGEs and ROS are uniquely intertwined. For an AGE to be created inside the body, the protein or the fat that creates the bond has to be oxidized first, usually by ROS. Therefore, having higher ROS levels means having more AGEs. Once an AGE is created, the damage and inflammation it causes results in the formation of more ROS, and a negative cycle is established.

AGEs and the damage they cause are now linked to cellular aging and premature aging inside the body and in various organs. Over a dozen different AGEs have been identified in the human body, and about half are known to accumulate with age in skin cells, affecting collagen production and promoting wrinkling and thinning of the skin. The rest of the AGEs can start accumulating in other organs and in the bloodstream, causing aging and cellular damage in the heart and cardiovascular system, kidneys, liver, and brain, resulting in chronic age-related diseases in these organs.

The link between AGEs and age-related diseases was recognized as early as 2001, when medical researchers at the University of South Carolina reported in the journal *Experimental Gerontology* that "they [AGEs] accumulate to high levels in tissues in age-related chronic diseases, such as atherosclerosis, diabetes, arthritis and neurodegenerative disease. Inhibition of AGE formation in these diseases may limit oxidative and inflammatory damage in tissues, retarding the progression of pathophysiology and improve the quality of life during aging." Recently, measuring AGE levels in individuals over age 60 has been proposed as a possible new blood test to monitor healthy aging and to enable the early detection of age-related diseases.

Methylglyoxal (MG) is one of the most reactive glycating agents, which results in the formation of advanced glycation end products (AGEs). AGEs have been implicated in the progression of age-related diseases in humans. Research conducted in 2015 by researchers in Thailand revealed that chanca piedra could significantly reduce the formation of MG-derived AGEs *in vitro*. Another research group in India tested chanca piedra and one of the plant's main active chemicals, phyllanthin, for AGE-inhibitor actions and published their research in the same year. The reported that *in vitro*, 100 micrograms of chanca piedra inhibited the formation of AGEs by over 78 percent. In administering the plant and the extracted chemical to mice, they also reported strong ant-AGE actions that were better than the other plants and chemicals they tested in comparison. Both of these research groups attributed the AGE-inhibiting actions of chanca piedra, at least in part, to the strong antioxidant actions and high amounts of polyphenols this plant provides. Another study confirmed chanca piedra's ability to lower AGE levels and AGE damage in diabetic animals in 2011.

A patent was awarded in 2015 and assigned to Johnson & Johnson Consumer Companies, Inc. on an extraction method for chanca piedra, which extracted the polyphenols and anti-AGE active chemicals for the plant. Their claims in the patent was that their chanca piedra extract was suitable for topical use to reduce skin aging and AGE levels in the skin.

Antidiabetic & Cholesterol Lowering Actions

Type 2 diabetes is categorized as a chronic inflammatory disease that is associated with oxidative stress and insulin resistance. The increased production of reactive oxygen species (ROS) or a reduced capacity of the ROS-scavenging antioxidants can lead to abnormal changes in intracellular signaling and result in chronic inflammation and insulin resistance. Prevention of ROS-induced oxidative stress and inflammation can be an important therapeutic strategy to prevent the onset of type 2 diabetes and well as diabetic complications and co-occurring diseases. Chanca piedra's strong antioxidant and cellular-protective antioxidant actions previously discussed in this chapter will be beneficial to people with type 2 diabetes. Several of the studies discussed in chanca piedra's cellular-protective antioxidant actions were conducted on diabetic animals. Chanca piedra was able to protect the kidney, pancreas, and heart from the normal damage diabetes causes to these organs.

Chanca piedra's AGE-inhibiting actions also provides important information for diabetics. The initiation and progression of diabetes can also be linked to higher AGE levels in the body and the cellular damage, generation of additional free radicals, and inflammation these AGEs cause. Diabetics have much higher levels of both AGEs and ROS, and the cellular damage caused by both are strongly associated with the development of other diabetic complications like high blood pressure and cholesterol levels, macular degeneration, diabetic neuropathy, fatty liver, and kidney damage leading to renal failure.

Chanca piedra and several closely related *Phyllanthus* plant species have been used in Ayurvedic medicine in India for diabetes for more than 2,000 years. In addition to the antioxidant, cellular- protective, and AGE-inhibiting actions, the plants have shown in animal research to lower blood sugar levels. These include early animal studies published in 1982, 1995, 2001, 2002, 2006, and 2008 by researchers in India and Southeast Asia.

Another early study in 1989 reported that chanca piedra has aldose reductase inhibitory properties. The Indian researchers studying chanca piedra's AGE-inhibiting actions in 2015 also confirmed the plant's ability to inhibit this enzyme. Aldose reductase is an enzyme involved in carbohydrate metabolism that converts sugar (glucose) to sorbitol. The enzyme acts on nerve endings exposed to a high concentration of blood sugar and thus may lead to many diabetic complications, such as diabetic neuropathy and macular degeneration. Substances that inhibit the enzyme can prevent some of the chemical imbalances that occur and thus protect the nerves from the risk of developing such complications.

Increased oxidative stress due to chronic high blood sugar is a widely accepted factor in the progression of diabetes and its complications. Animal studies using chanca piedra have demonstrated dose-dependent improvements in fasting blood sugar, improved glucose tolerance, and restoration of pancreatic tissue architecture, which may be due to inhibition of enzymatic pathways in intestinal carbohydrate digestion and glucose storage. It is thought that the active compounds in the plant possess insulin-mimicking activity or potentially may stimulate the production of insulin in the liver as observed by the plant's beneficial effects on liver enzyme levels. Despite these findings, the antidiabetic activity of chanca piedra remains uncertain with varying results from different members of the genus. Once again, better results were reported for the South American *Phyllanthus niruri* species than the Indian and Asian species of *Phyllanthus amarus*. However, more studies were conducted on the *amarus* species than the *niruri* species.

The animal and *in vitro* studies conducted on the *niruri* species of chanca piedra have concluded that the plant's antidiabetic actions have several mechanisms of actions. First, chanca piedra has plant compounds that interfere with two digestive enzymes (alpha-amylase and alpha-glucosidase) that break down sugars and starches during digestion. When these enzymes are inhibited, the starches and sugars in a meal are not broken down to enable absorption (which subsequently raises blood sugar levels) and are eliminated in the stool instead. This action was tested *in vitro* and in animals in six different research studies, and researchers suggested that chanca piedra's ability to lower blood sugar levels were probably due in large part to these digestive enzyme–inhibitor compounds. When chanca piedra was tested *in vitro*, it inhibited alpha-amylase in dosages of only 2 milligrams, and alpha-glucosidase in smaller dosages of only 200 micrograms. Other enzyme inhibitor studies on *Phyllanthus amarus* required significantly higher dosages to achieve the same inhibitory activity.

The next helpful mechanism of action with regard to diabetes is chanca piedra's well-studied ability to improve liver function. The liver stores and releases insulin as the body needs it, and recent research with diabetic animals reports that chanca piedra can improve the liver's ability to store and release insulin more effectively. It is believed that the plant's lowering effect on free radicals and AGEs is having a positive effect on the liver, enabling it to perform this essential function and maintain better insulin levels.

Newer research in 2019 reports that chanca piedra can have a beneficial effect on leptin levels, which directly affect diabetes. Leptin is a natural pro-inflammatory compound we produce mainly in our fat cells. Leptin controls insulin sensitivity levels (as well as appetite). When our fat cells increase as we gain weight, leptin levels rise and our bodies can quickly become leptin resistant. This then causes most of our cells to start losing sensitivity to insulin, requiring more and more insulin to produce the same effect and taxing the pancreas to increase output of insulin. High leptin levels also generate a great deal of chronic inflammation in our body fat and other internal organs, including the brain. The researchers in this recent research suggested that chanca piedra's ability to restore leptin levels to healthy levels contributed to better insulin sensitivity for type 2 diabetics, which has a "side effect" of lowering blood sugar levels.

Several human studies attempting to prove clinically the antidiabetic potency of chanca piedra and its closely related other species have also been conducted, even though the results were not consistent with each other in terms of the hypoglycemic activity of the genus. Nor did the human studies always re-create the results achieved in animals.

A clinical study that evaluated several effects (i.e., diuretic, hypotensive, and hypoglycemic effects of

Phyllanthus amarus) was conducted in 1995. Nine individuals with mild hypertension (four also with diabetes mellitus) were treated with a preparation of the whole plant of *Phyllanthus amarus* for 10 days. They reported a significant increase in 24-hour urine volume, and urine and serum sodium levels was observed. A significant reduction of systolic blood pressure in nondiabetic hypertensives and female subjects was noted. And blood sugar levels were also significantly reduced in the entire group treated with chanca piedra. However, the study sample size was too small to draw an adequate conclusion, including regarding its direct blood sugar–lowering effect. No control group was allocated in the study.

Quite a different finding was reported in another crossover clinical study published in 2001. In the study, researchers evaluated the glycemic response of 21 patients with non-insulin-dependent diabetes mellitus given 100 milliliters of a water extract from 12.5 grams of powdered *Phyllanthus amarus* twice daily. They reported no hypoglycemic actions after one week. To date, no human diabetes studies have been conducted on the *niruri* species, which has much higher levels of AGE-inhibitor and enzyme inhibitor compounds than the *amarus* species has.

Diuretic Actions

Chanca piedra has a long history of use in traditional medicine system around the world as an effective herbal diuretic. Various human and animal studies conducted on chanca piedra's ability to treat kidney stones reported that urine output was moderately to significantly increased in their research. Other researchers reported that chanca piedra's ability to reduce blood pressure in animals was at least partially attributed to the plant's diuretic abilities, which they also noted in their studies. In 2010, researchers in India gave rats a water extract of chanca piedra and reported that it was almost as effective as a standard diuretic drug (hydrochlorothiazide) for increasing urination. Several other studies also confirm a similar diuretic effect with *Phyllanthus amarus*. See the reference section for a listing of this research on chanca piedra's diuretic actions.

Benefits and Actions for the Heart

Chanca piedra was first reported to lower blood pressure in laboratory animals by researchers in India in 1982. They were actually studying the herb's ability to lower blood sugar levels and reported lowered blood pressure as a side effect. Since that time, several other researchers have made the same observations while studying other aspects of chanca piedra. Most recently, Brazilian researchers studying patients with kidney stones reported in 2018 that it effectively lowered their blood pressure levels (while treating their stones).

Several research groups have specifically studied chanca piedra's ability to lower blood pressure in animals over the years. Indian researchers studied rats with diabetes and hypertension in 2016. They gave the animals a water extract of chanca piedra and reported that it provided a significant decrease in blood pressure and a decrease in liver enzyme levels as well as better blood sugar levels. They reported that their study supported the traditional use of chanca piedra for diabetes and hypertension and stated that it "may have a beneficial effect in patients with co-existing diabetic hypertension." Most recently, Malaysian researchers studied chanca piedra in rats with hypertension in 2020 and reported that a water extract of chanca piedra effectively lowered blood pressure in animals by providing vasorelaxant and vasodilator actions. Other researchers in Africa reported the same hypotensive actions of *Phyllanthus amarus* in rabbits in 2013.

Several research groups have been studying which natural compounds in chanca piedra might be responsible for the plant's ability to lower blood pressure. Thus far, phyllanthin, hypophyllanthin, geraniin, and methyl brevifolincarboxylate have demonstrated vasodilator, vasorelaxant, and/or ACE-inhibitor actions in animal and test-tube research.

In addition to lowering blood pressure, chanca piedra's strong antioxidant actions have been shown to protect the heart. Two studies were published in 2011 and 2019, which reported that chanca piedra could protect the heart from damage caused by a common heart-toxic chemotherapy drug called doxorubicin. One group gave animals chanca piedra while they administered the chemo drug, and the other group pretreated the animals with chanca piedra before administering the drug. Both reported that the antioxidant actions of the herb prevented the normal damage to the heart that was observed in the control group (the animals given the drug without chanca piedra). Both research groups suggested that chanca piedra could be a therapeutic agent for the treatment of cardiovascular complications associated with known heart-toxic pharmaceutical drugs.

Another research group studied chanca piedra's ability to protect the heart in animals that were fed a high-fructose diet. Fructose significantly elevates free radicals, which can be damaging to the heart, veins, and arteries, and oxidizes more cholesterol, which can deposit in the heart and veins. These Indian researchers reported in 2017 that chanca piedra protected the hearts of rats from the negative effects of high levels of fructose, increased natural antioxidant chemicals in the heart and aorta, prevented cell death, decreased cholesterol levels, and reduced fatty deposits in the heart and veins.

Chanca piedra's ability to lower blood pressure generates one of the precautions and possible drug interactions listed for the plant in the consumer guide in the next chapter. People who are already taking antihypertensive drugs for high blood pressure should monitor their blood pressure levels regularly when they first take chanca piedra to determine what kind of effect this natural remedy has on their heart, as medications may need to be adjusted. Whenever you are taking prescription drugs, including blood pressure drugs, it's always best to check with your healthcare provider before taking any herbal remedy.

Other Areas of Study

Two animal studies report that using chanca piedra topically and taking it internally speeds the healing of burns and wounds. Other researchers have reported that chanca piedra may be a beneficial for osteoporosis. In addition to its confirmed anti-inflammatory actions, researchers published two studies in 2018 and 2019 that one of chanca piedra's active compounds (geraniin) was capable *in vitro* and in rodents to modulate a biochemical process that results in bone loss in people and animals with osteoporosis. Lastly, recent research on chanca piedra suggests it might promote hair growth. Five studies have been published between 2014 and 2019 by researchers in India and Indonesia that reports chanca piedra increased the growth of hair in animals. One of these studies reported that chanca piedra protected rats from the hair loss normally caused by a chemotherapy drug (doxorubicin).

Summary

With more than 130 active compounds found in chanca piedra, it's not all that surprising that it has a great deal of varied benefits, uses, and actions. Some of the benefits in various diseases and conditions are provided by the 70-plus polyphenols effectively relieving stress and damage caused by free radicals. I was amazed at all the new research that has been conducted on chanca piedra since I wrote about in my last two rainforest books. Most of the new research continues to validate chanca piedra for the majority of its traditional uses in herbal medicine, as well as reports a few new uses. Chanca piedra has long been my go-to herb for most all urinary and liver issues. All this new research just explains why it's worked so well for so many years.

CHAPTER 6

A Consumer Guide for Chanca Piedra

If you have read the earlier chapters of this book, you may be ready to purchase the first chanca piedra product that you find online or in a store. However, before you make that purchase, there are a few important factors of which you should be aware. Over the years, I have found that when a nutritional supplement becomes popular, the market is flooded with dozens of products marketed under the name of that substance. Unfortunately, just because a product bears the name "chanca piedra" doesn't mean that it is a high-quality supplement which contains all of the chemical compounds that make it an effective herbal remedy. Some products haven't been properly tested for chemical compounds, some haven't been processed properly, and some may not even contain the right plant!

In this chapter, we will look at the most important issues you should consider when buying chanca piedra so that you get the most effective product on the market.

Traditional Preparation

In traditional medicine systems around the world, chanca piedra is most commonly prepared as a standard herbal infusion when it is harvested fresh. Basically, making an infusion is similar to preparing a cup of hot tea. One tablespoon of cut-up fresh chanca piedra whole herb is placed into a coffee cup or mug and boiling water is poured over the herb. It is allowed to steep for 10 minutes. The herb is then strained out, and the infusion is consumed, usually twice daily.

When dried chanca piedra herb is used, it is prepared as a decoction. One teaspoon of the dried tea-cut or one teaspoon of the dried herb powder is placed in a pot with a cup of water, and it is boiled gently for 10 minutes. Strain the cut herb out of the decoction and pour into a mug. If you are using a powdered whole herb, the powder will settle to the bottom of the pan and you can simply pour the decoction off the top and into a mug.

Chanca piedra's active natural compounds are water soluble, so this traditional preparation is confirmed to be effective through scientific research. This also indicates that you can substitute chanca piedra capsules or tablets for the tea as well. If it's easily extracted in water, it will be easily extracted during digestion.

The Safety of Chanca Piedra

The safety profile and tolerability of chanca piedra are based on available safety data and adverse events recorded in some of the clinical studies discussed in this chapter in this book. In every clinical study performed to date in humans, chanca piedra was well tolerated and no signs of toxicity or side effects were reported. Much the same was reported in the many animal studies performed on chanca piedra and other related *Phyllanthus* species. Furthermore, a phase 1 clinical study of a *Phyllanthus* extract specifically aimed to evaluate the safety and tolerability of a formulated *Phyllanthus* extract in healthy subjects was also conducted in 2004. Chanca piedra was also studied in children as young as four years of age, and no clinically significant adverse events were found during the study course. See the reference section for a listing of the safety studies conducted. All in all, the research report the safety of chanca piedra is quite good, it's well tolerated by both animals and humans, and few if any side effects were noted.

■ CONSIDERATIONS

Chanca piedra is a very powerful medicinal plant with many active natural compounds, and research reveals that it can positively affect many diseases, organs, and system. As such, there are a few things to be aware of before you start taking chanca piedra. It is always important to be aware of the effects a supplement may have on your body. Whether you choose to take chanca piedra for kidney stones or infections, or for another medicinal use, you should keep the following considerations in mind:

- ❑ Based on studies with diabetic animals, chanca piedra may affect blood sugar levels. If you have diabetes and take diabetic medications, test your sugar levels more often than usual until you determine what effects chanca piedra is having on your blood sugar. Your diabetes medications may need to be adjusted when using chanca piedra. Continue to monitor your blood sugar levels as long as you are taking chanca piedra. Some of the plant's documented benefits for diabetes can have a cumulative effect by increasing insulin sensitivity. If you have diabetes, always check with your doctor prior to taking any new herbal supplement.

- ❑ If you are taking a statin drug to manage your cholesterol, have your cholesterol levels checked by your doctor if you use chanca piedra for longer than three months. Animal studies indicate that chanca piedra can lower cholesterol levels, and your medications may need to be adjusted.

- ❑ Several research studies on chanca piedra in animals and humans reported that chanca piedra can lower blood pressure. If you are under the care of a physician for hypertension and take antihypertensive drugs, always check with your doctor prior to taking any new herbal supplement. Monitor your blood pressure levels much more often when you begin using chanca piedra. Your high blood pressure medications may need to be adjusted when using chanca piedra.

- ❑ Several studies reported that chanca piedra has a diuretic action and increases urination. If you are already taking diuretic drugs, using chanca piedra might potentiate or increase the actions of these drugs, and your medications may need to be adjusted. Check with your doctor before taking chanca piedra if you are currently using diuretics.

■ CONTRAINDICATIONS AND POSSIBLE DRUG INTERACTIONS

The following contraindications and cautions are based on traditional uses and animal studies and may not specifically relate to human consumption. However, it is always best to err on the side of caution, especially since more often than not, traditional uses are eventually confirmed by research.

Contraindications

- ❑ Chanca piedra has been used traditionally as a menstrual stimulant. Women who are pregnant should always check with their doctor before taking any herbal supplement. Since chanca piedra has not been studied in pregnant animals or humans, it is contraindicated in pregnancy.
- ❑ If you have low blood pressure or low blood sugar (hypoglycemia), it is best to avoid using chanca piedra.

Possible Drug Interactions

- ❑ Based on animal research and a few human studies, chanca piedra may enhance the effects of drugs taken to lower blood sugar, cholesterol levels, and blood pressure. If you are taking medications for these conditions, speak to your doctor before taking chanca piedra, and be sure to have your doctor monitor you during the first month of chanca piedra use.
- ❑ Test-tube (in vitro) research published in 2011 suggests that chanca piedra inhibits an enzyme called CYP3A4. This have not been confirmed in animals or humans yet,

but it is best to err on the side of caution. This enzyme is found in the intestines and liver and is mainly responsible for metabolizing drugs. It is not unusual for polyphenol-rich medicinal plants and even fruit juices to have enzyme inhibitor actions—including inhibiting this particular enzyme. For example, grapefruit juice is a powerful inhibitor of CYP3A4. When taken with grapefruit juice, drugs metabolized by CYP3A4 have a higher bioavailability and therefore may have a higher risk of adverse effects. If you are taking any prescription drug, ask your doctor if CYP3A4-inhibitors will react with any drug they have prescribed to you. Again, this has not been proven in humans, but it's better to be cautious and know what to watch for in possible drug-herb interactions.

There is rarely enough scientific research performed on natural health remedies to determine their effects in combination with the many drugs that are commonly prescribed today. If you have any condition for which you have been prescribed a medication, it is always best to check with your doctor before trying any new herbal supplement or natural remedy.

Finding a Good Chanca Piedra Product

The first thing to determine when looking for available chanca piedra products is to determine where the plant came from. The true *Phyllanthus niruri* species of chanca piedra is only available to U.S. manufacturers from harvesting programs in Peru and Brazil. Most of it is wild harvested or wild cultivated with very few actual cultivation programs established to date. Most U.S. manufacturers of chanca piedra herbal supplements will say on their label, marketing materials, or website where their chanca piedra was harvested.

Suppliers from India and China are selling bulk supplies of "chanca piedra" to U.S. manufacturers and even calling it *Phyllanthus niruri* in some instances. However, this species is not native to India or China. *Phyllanthus amarus* is usually the real species sold as *niruri* from these countries. However, even then, other *Phyllanthus* native species may be adulterating their products. In India, *Phyllanthus amarus* is sold under the trade name *Bhumyamalaki*. During a market surveillance of herbal drugs conducted in 2006, researchers reported that they observed that almost all the commercial samples they tested were either comprised of *Phyllanthus amarus* and *Phyllanthus maderaspatensis*. Or they contained a mixture of *Phyllanthus amarus, Phyllanthus fraternus,* and *Phyllanthus maderaspatensis*. These researchers also reported that *Phyllanthus amarus* was the only species of the three that actually contained two main active compounds in chanca piedra, which provides a wide variety of benefits: phyllanthin and hypophyllanthin. The same problem exists in China since they have 18 different native species of *Phyllanthus* plants, and *niruri* is not one of them. *Phyllanthus urinaria* is the most widely sold species in China, and it is often exported to the United States as *Phyllanthus niruri*.

The *niruri* and *amarus* species are the closest related when it comes to their plant chemistry. Both contain the main active natural compounds that have been researched with biological actions; the *amarus* species just contain less of those compounds than *niruri* does. If you look at the animal research (and both species have been well studied in animals), they both seem to work equally for some things, but *niruri* seems to be a much better antiviral and antimicrobial. The *niruri* species does contain a handful of natural compounds that are absent in the *amarus* species as well.

For all of these reasons, it's better to find a product that contains chanca piedra that came from Brazil or Peru. If it doesn't say so on the label, ask questions.

Choosing the Best Form of Chanca Piedra

Currently, there are several different types of chanca piedra products sold in the United States. They include capsules, tablets, and liquid extracts, as well as bulk powdered chanca piedra herb, tea bags, and loose tea-cut herb, which is sold by the ounce or by the pound. Dry 4:1 extracts are also sold in capsules or in bulk. The forms discussed next include those that are currently available as well as those that may be offered over time.

Capsules and Tablets

Chanca piedra is available under various labels that offer either tablets or capsules. Since the main active compounds in chanca piedra are water soluble, they'll be easily digested and absorbed when taking capsules or tablets. Other than buying the plant in bulk and preparing infusions/tea, this is the easiest method to take chanca piedra with the best benefits. Make sure the name in the "Supplement Facts" says *Phyllanthus niruri*.

Liquid Extracts

Many medicinal plants are prepared as liquid extracts. The plant is simply soaked in a liquid, which usually consists of water and alcohol or water and glycerin. Extracts are most commonly prepared by soaking one part plant in four parts liquid, which is a higher concentration than you would use to prepare a tea. Once the plant has soaked for a time—between 5 and 30 days, depending on the plant and the manufacturer—the plant is strained out, and the liquid is filtered and bottled.

Unfortunately, you can never be sure which compounds are released from the plant and remain in the extract and which are thrown away when the plant is strained out. Actual compound extraction in these products can vary widely, depending on the liquid used and the compounds' reaction to the liquid.

Liquid extracts are thought to be an efficient means of getting a plant's active ingredients into the bloodstream quickly. As a liquid, an extract is absorbed through the tissues in the mouth, throat, and on its way down to the stomach, avoiding much of the digestive process.

Liquid extracts are thought to be more concentrated than herbal teas, so the dosages are lower than that of teas—usually around 1 to 2 milliliters. However, as mentioned earlier, the extract may not contain the specific compounds that you want and need. The following discussions of tinctures and glycerin-based extracts—the two types of liquid extracts employed for most medicinal plants—explain why some important compounds may be missing from these products.

Tinctures

Herbal remedies are often prepared as liquid extracts called tinctures, which have been used in herbal medicine for centuries. A tincture is prepared by soaking the plant in a combination of water and alcohol for a period of time. The concept is that the active compounds will dissolve or be extracted into the liquid as the plant soaks in the solution. The plant is then strained out of the extract and thrown away, and the tincture is filtered and bottled. The alcohol acts as a preservative so that the tincture can be stored for a longer period of time.

This technique works well for some medicinal plants, but not all of them. Too often, manufacturers ignore the unique chemistry of each plant and employ the same method for all species. If the plant has delicate water-soluble chemicals and compounds as chanca piedra has, they can be damaged or degraded in alcohol, and they simply won't be present in the resulting tincture. The research on chanca piedra's antiviral actions confirms the problem of what happens when an extract method leaves behind important plant chemicals. Over many years, water extracts of chanca piedra were demonstrated to have much better antiviral actions against hepatitis viruses than alcohol extracts did.

The number and ratio of active compounds will always be different in a tincture than in the natural plant, simply because medicinal plants have so many different compounds that may or may not be extracted by the method used. Because a full chemical analysis is very expensive to perform, manufacturers rarely, if ever, test finished tincture products to determine which compounds are present. Keep in mind that there are over 100 hundred different active compounds in chanca piedra. Determining if every compound is present in a tincture—and, if so, how much is present—would take a great deal of time and cost a great deal of money.

Glycerin-Based Liquid Extracts

A relative newcomer to herbal medicine is the water extract of a plant that uses glycerin instead of alcohol as a preservative. This came about as an alternative for children, animals, and adults when palatability and alcohol sensitivities are primary considerations. The food-grade vegetable glycerin used is extracted from vegetable oils. Sometimes referred to as glycerol, it is a clear, colorless, and odorless liquid with an incredibly sweet taste and the consistency of a thick syrup.

Glycerin doesn't greatly aid in the extraction of plant compounds. It is mostly used as a preservative in herbal extracts to extend their shelf life. Although glycerin is less effective than alcohol as a preservative, smart and ethical manufacturers use this extraction method for plants with delicate water-soluble plant compounds. When I was manufacturing rainforest herbal products, I offered chanca piedra in capsules and in a water-glycerin liquid extract and never as a tincture.

Concentrated Dry Extracts

Today, dry extracts of medicinal plants are quite popular in the U.S. health products industry. Several concentrated dry extracts of chanca piedra are sold in the American natural products market, but personally, I don't recommend them.

The goal of these products is to "condense and concentrate" the plant so that less is supposedly needed to get the same benefits. What 4-to-1 really means is that when the manufacturer began the process, it had four parts of the original plant material, and at the end of the process, it was "condensed" to just one part. You'll see these products marketed as "four times as strong" as the natural plant. In other words, one pound of the extract is equal to four pounds of the plant, so supposedly you can take a lesser amount to achieve the same results. Unfortunately, most of the time, these statements are neither true nor accurate.

The dry extract process might work for some types of plants, but it doesn't work for all of them—and it certainly doesn't work for chanca piedra. Why? This process usually starts by making an alcohol tincture, which is then spray dried under high heat. As we learned in the discussion of tinctures, chanca piedra doesn't much like alcohol, and many of the delicate water-soluble chemicals degrade or disappear. Therefore, this process causes some beneficial compounds to be lost completely—not to be present at four times their natural concentration.

In addition, what you'll rarely see on the label of these products is that just before these tinctures are spray dried, they are mixed with a lot of sugar. Dextrose is the main sugar used in the United States, but anything can be used in China, including corn syrup. Sugar is added to thicken the tincture and to provide the bulk needed to hold on to the extracted compounds. As a result, 50 percent or more of these finished spray-dried extracts are actually some form of sugar, yet the label just says "4:1 Concentrated Extract."

Personally, I've never been a fan of concentrated

spray-dried extracts. I believe that the active compounds found in medicinal plants are too important to ignore and are the main reason we take them to improve our health. I want to know that the active compounds—which have been scientifically confirmed to have specific actions—are actually present in the product I am taking. I am definitely not alone in that belief, which is why standardized extracts were created. These products, however, aren't perfect either.

Standardized Extracts

Standardized extracts usually employ extraction through alcohol as already described, but they guarantee that the resulting extract has one or more compounds present in specific amounts, usually expressed as a percentage. Manufacturers can use other drastic chemicals instead of alcohol to obtain the desired compounds, but they usually don't state their extraction method or which chemicals they used. Unlike spray-dried concentrated extracts—which never provide a chemical analysis of what they actually extracted—these products at least test and guarantee a certain amount of one or more beneficial compounds in the product they sell.

When you end up extracting some compounds but not others, and/or you change the ratio of the compounds that are present, you lose the synergy that nature put in these plants. Many natural plant compounds interact with one another, working together to create greater benefits than the sum of their separate benefits. Some natural compounds can actually bind together and create an entirely new compound that has beneficial actions greater than those of the individual unbound compounds. (Polyphenols are well known to do this regularly.) This has been scientifically demonstrated time and time again with many medicinal plants, including chanca piedra.

With over 100 active compounds in a plant like chanca piedra, we just aren't smart enough to determine how all these active chemicals are working synergistically together. More important, the reason herbal remedies—full of many active compounds—can heal without the side effects associated with single-chemical drugs is that the interaction of all those natural chemicals often mitigate any adverse effects. Standardized extracts may have a standardized amount of a particular chemical or group of chemicals, but the remaining beneficial chemicals that occur in the natural plant vary greatly in these products.

Several standardized extracts of chanca piedra are sold in other countries, including India, Malaysia, and Indonesia. It is possible one or more of these standardized extracts might show up here in the U.S. market sometime in the future. Again, I don't recommend them. Most of these are standardized to contain "10% tannins," and some say they're using *P. niruri* while others (more accurately) say they're using *P. amarus*. Tannins are a type of polyphenol, but there are many other beneficial compounds in this rainforest plant that are not tannins, including beneficial flavonoids, alkaloids, saponins, and other active compounds. But let's look at a real comparison. Natural chanca piedra whole herb naturally contains around 7.5 percent tannins. It's much cheaper to use a teaspoon of chanca piedra powder to make a cup of tea and get 375 milligrams of tannins than to take a 500-milligram capsule of standardized extract to get 50 milligrams of tannins. And, with a cup of natural tea, you're getting all the compounds (and non-tannin active chemicals) that nature put in the plant and not just those chemicals that were extracted in a complicated proprietary man-made process that left some behind.

The bottom line is this: Nature is a much better chemist than humans. In chanca piedra, nature has provided dozens of compounds that work together to provide great health benefits. Since chanca piedra and its compounds are easily digested, personally, I'll stick with the whole-herb powder and take it in capsules or tablets or just prepare a tea with it.

Where to Purchase Chanca Piedra

Chanca piedra products are sold under various brand names and are available in health food stores and through many online retailers. Chanca piedra can also be found as an ingredient in various herbal formulas, including formulas to support the liver, kidneys, and herbal antiviral formulas. See the resource section for more information on the products I personally purchase now for myself and family. Just remember to look for a product made with plants harvested in South America, and choose a whole herb instead of extracted herb product for the best results.

Conclusion

Chanca piedra has been my go-to herb for more than 20 years for kidney stones, gout, gallstones, viral infections, and liver diseases. I hope you've learned why after reading this book. In fact, if I had to choose a single herb (and no other) for these particular five conditions, I would choose chanca piedra—without question. I was quite interested to see that this rainforest remedy has new scientific validation on its possible uses for high blood pressure, diabetes, and lowering cholesterol. However, over the last year, I've read thousands and thousands of studies on the benefits and actions of plant polyphenol compounds being highly beneficial for these three purposes, so I'm really not surprised. Chanca piedra delivers an incredible amount of well-studied, as well as, novel polyphenols with many health benefits and actions.

The most important takeaway for me in reading several hundred studies on chanca piedra and other closely related *Phyllanthus* herbs in order to write this book is the real possibility to use chanca piedra for the current coronavirus we're all facing presently as well as others that might emerge in the future. I don't know today if chanca piedra can kill this particular coronavirus outright like it can other viruses. That it boosts the immune system to fight both bacterial and viral infections naturally, as well as lowers inflammatory cytokines to protect the lungs from inflammation and cell damage that bacteria and virus causes in the lungs, was enough for me to stock up on chanca piedra to protect myself and family, just in case, during these current trying times.

I sincerely hope that researchers will test this remarkable rainforest plant for this coronavirus to determine not only if it can kill the virus outright or just inhibit its growth, but also if it can be beneficial to modulate the immune system to help the body fight the virus naturally and protect the lungs simultaneously, as was demonstrated in tuberculosis and asthma patients studied in the past. The absolute safety, lack of side effects, and overall great tolerance reported in all the human studies conducted on chanca piedra thus far should be a compelling reason to further study this remarkable rainforest medicinal herb in humans with viral infections as quickly as possible. Amidst the current chaos, one can only hope at this point.

Maybe, just maybe, this book will get into the right hands to make this a reality, especially in developing tropical nations where chanca piedra grows naturally to provide a locally sourced, cost-effective natural remedy for these life-threatening emerging viruses. Even China has their own native species of very similar *Phyllanthus* herbs with almost as many of the same antiviral natural plant compounds found in chanca piedra . . . maybe they'll be the first. Doctors is China are certainly more open to plant-based drugs and remedies than American doctors are. I'll be watching and ready to report, just in case.

In the meantime, I have set up a page for chanca piedra

on my personal blog at https://leslie-taylor-raintree.blogspot.com where I'll post any updates if they come available. If you end up using chanca piedra to treat this current coronavirus, please take the time to post your experience and results; it's important information to share with all. Also feel free to ask questions and share your experiences using chanca piedra for any other uses on this blog page as well.

Resources

Where I Buy Bulk Rainforest Plants
(by the pound or kilogram)

Nutricargo: Clifton, NJ 07011 • (866) 371-0779 • www.nutricargo.com

Amazon Discovery: Tamaqua, PA 18252 • (855) 766-1772 • www.amazondiscovery.com

Where I Buy Rainforest Herbal Supplements

Rainforest Pharmacy: Miami, FL 33177 • (305) 235-9880 • www.rainpharm.com

HOW TO PREPARE RAINFOREST FORMULAS

I discussed several rainforest formulas in this book that I developed and used for many years, including Amazon A-V for viruses, Amazon Kidney Support for kidney stones, Amazon Urinary Support for urinary tract infections, Amazon KDY-CL for kidney support and regeneration, and Amazon Gallbladder Support for gallstones and sluggish bile.

The main ingredient in all these formulas is chanca piedra. More information on these rainforest herbal formulas is available online at www.rain-tree.com/rtmprod.htm. More information on the rainforest plants in these formulas can be found in the Tropical Plant Database online at www.rain-tree.com/plants.htm. Some of these formulas may be available from other manufacturers who copied my formula directions on the Rain-Tree website.

To prepare these formulas yourself, follow these instructions:

♦ Amazon A-V

A combination of rainforest plants with antiviral actions

A blend of chanca piedra, bitter melon, clavillia, mullaca, jergon sacha, carqueja, amargo, mutamba, and anamu

Directions: To prepare this natural remedy, use one equal part of each plant listed. To make a small amount, "one part" could be 1 tablespoon (you'd have 9 tablespoons of the blended herbal formula). For larger amounts, "one part" could be 1 ounce or 1 cup or 1 pound. Combine all the herbs together well. The herbal mixture can then be stuffed into capsules or brewed into tea or stirred into juice or other liquid.

Suggested use: Take 2 grams three times daily (1 gram is about $^1/_2$ teaspoon by volume).

Contraindications: Not to be used during pregnancy or while breastfeeding.

Drug interactions: None reported.

Other practitioner observations: Several ingredients in this formula have demonstrated antibacterial actions, which might reduce friendly bacteria in the stomach and intestines. Supplementing the diet with probiotics and digestive enzymes is advisable if this formula is used for longer than 30 days.

♦ Amazon Kidney Support

A combination of rainforest plants used for kidney stones

A blend of chanca piedra, boldo, erva tostão, cipó cabeludo, and abuta

Directions: To prepare this natural remedy, use four parts chanca piedra, two parts boldo, erva tostão, and cipó cabeludo, and one part abuta. To make a small amount, "one part" could be 1 tablespoon (you'd have 11 tablespoons of the blended herbal formula). For larger amounts, "one part" could be 1 ounce or 1 cup or 1 pound. Combine all the herbs together well. The herbal mixture can then be stuffed into capsules or brewed into tea or stirred into juice or other liquid.

Suggested use: Take 1 to 2 grams three times daily (1 gram is about $^1/_2$ teaspoon by volume).

Contraindications: Not to be used during pregnancy or while breastfeeding.

Drug interactions: May increase the potency of diabetic, heart, anticoagulant, and diuretic medications.

Other practitioner observations: 1) Several plants in this formula have been documented to reduce blood pressure and/or have a mild cardiac depressant effect in animal studies. Individuals with low blood pressure should be monitored for this possible effect; 2) Several plants in this formula contain coumarin, which thins the blood. Individuals with blood disorders such as hemophilia should be monitored closely for this possible effect; and, 3)Plants in this formula have a diuretic activity. Chronic long-term use of any diuretic can cause electrolyte and mineral imbalances, which should be monitored more closely.

♦ Amazon Urinary Support

A combination of rainforest plants used for urinary tract infections

A blend of chanca piedra, anamu, jatoba, Brazilian peppertree, pau d'arco, erva tostão, and guaco

Directions: To prepare this natural remedy, use three parts chanca piedra, two parts anamu, jatoba, Brazilian peppertree, and pau d'arco, and one part each of erva tostão and guaco. To make a small amount, "one part" could be 1 tablespoon (you'd have 13 tablespoons of the blended herbal formula). For larger amounts, "one part" could be 1 ounce or 1 cup or 1 pound. Combine all the herbs together well. The herbal mixture can then be stuffed into capsules or brewed into tea or stirred into juice or other liquid.

Suggested use: Take 1.5 to 2 grams three times daily (1 gram is approximately $^1/_2$ teaspoon by volume).

Contraindications: Not to be used during pregnancy or while breastfeeding.

Drug interactions: Based on animal studies, it may increase the potency of anticoagulants and antihypertensive drugs.

Other practitioner observations: 1) Several plants in this formula have been documented to reduce blood pressure in animal studies. Individuals with low blood pressure should be monitored for this possible effect; 2) Several ingredients in the formula have demonstrated antimicrobial activities in laboratory studies. Adding probiotics to the diet may be beneficial when this formula is used for longer than 30 days.

♦ Amazon KD-CL Support

A combination of rainforest plants to support and detox the kidneys during times of special needs (cirrhosis, dialysis, liver cancer, etc.)

A blend of chanca piedra, jatoba, anamu, matico, and amor seco

Directions: To prepare this natural remedy, use two parts chanca piedra and one part each of jatoba, anamu, matico, and amor seco. To make a small amount, "one part" could be 1 tablespoon (you'd have 6 tablespoons of the blended herbal formula). For larger amounts, "one part" could be 1 ounce or 1 cup or 1 pound. Combine all the herbs together well. The herbal mixture can then be stuffed into capsules or brewed into tea or stirred into juice or other liquid.

Suggested use: Take 1 to 2 grams twice daily (1 gram is approximately $^1/_2$ teaspoon by volume) or as directed by a health professional.

Contraindications: Not to be used during pregnancy or while breastfeeding.

Drug interactions: May increase the potency of antihypertensive and diuretic medications.

Other **practitioner observations**: 1) Several plants in this formula have been documented to reduce blood pressure in animal studies. Individuals with low blood pressure should be monitored for this possible effect; 2) Several plants in this formula have diuretic activity. Chronic long-term use of any diuretic can cause electrolyte and mineral imbalances, which should be monitored.

♦ Amazon Gallbladder Support

A combination of rainforest plants used for gallstones and sluggish bile

A blend of chanca piedra, artichoke, boldo, carqueja, erva tostão, condurango, gervâo, and jurubeba

Directions: To prepare this natural remedy, use three parts chanca piedra, two parts artichoke, and 1 part each of boldo, carqueja, erva tostão, condurango, gervâo, and jurubeba. To make a small amount, "one part" could be 1 tablespoon (you'd have 11 tablespoons of the blended herbal formula). For larger amounts, "one part" could be 1 ounce or 1 cup or 1 pound. Combine all the herbs together well. The herbal mixture can then be stuffed into capsules or brewed into tea or stirred into juice or other liquid.

Suggested use: Take 2 grams twice daily (by weight) (1 gram is approximately $^1/_2$ teaspoon by volume).

Contraindications: Not to be used during pregnancy, while breastfeeding, or while seeking to become pregnant.

Drug interactions: May increase the potency of antihypertensive, cholesterol and diabetic medications.

Other practitioner observations: 1) Several of the plants in this formula are documented with liver-detoxing actions, which may speed the clearance of drugs metabolized in the liver, thereby reducing their pharmacological effect or half-life; 2) Gervâo contains a small amount of salicylic acid. Those allergic or sensitive to aspirin or salicylates may wish to avoid this formula.

♦ Amazon Liver Support

Medicinal plants traditionally used in South America for liver cirrhosis, fatty liver, and other liver problems

A blend of chanca piedra, picão preto, carqueja, erva tostão, boldo, gervâo, fedegoso, and artichoke

Directions: To prepare this natural remedy, use three parts chanca piedra and one part each of picão preto, carqueja, erva tostão, boldo, gervâo, fedegoso, and artichoke. To make a small amount, "one part" could be 1 tablespoon (you'd have 10 tablespoons of the blended herbal formula). For larger amounts, "one part" could be 1 ounce or 1 cup or 1 pound. Combine all the herbs together well. The herbal mixture can then be stuffed into capsules or brewed into tea or stirred into juice or other liquid.

Suggested use: Take 2 grams two to three times daily (1 gram is about $^1/_2$ teaspoon by volume)

Contraindications: Not to be used during pregnancy or while breastfeeding.

Drug interactions: None reported; however, based on animal studies, it may increase the potency of antihypertensive drugs.

Other practitioner observations: 1) Several ingredients in the formula have been documented with liver-detoxing effects in animal studies. This may speed the clearance of some drugs metabolized in the liver (decrease the half-life), thereby reducing the pharmacological effect (and/or side effects) of certain drugs required to be metabolized in the liver. 2) Several plants in this formula have been documented to reduce blood pressure in animal studies. Individuals with low blood pressure should be monitored for this possible effect; and 3) Gervâo contains salicylic acid. Those allergic to aspirin or salicylates may wish to avoid this formula.

How to Add More Polyphenols to Your Diet

It's not that difficult to add high-polyphenol foods and beverages to your diet if you understand which fruits, vegetables, oils, grains, seeds, nuts, and beverages provide them. Phenol-Explorer is a great online resource that provides the polyphenol content of most common raw foods and beverages, as well as the content of the same foods processed or cooked using different methods. The searchable database contains 500 different polyphenols in more than 450 different foods. Access the polyphenol database online at http://phenol-explorer.eu/

References

This reference list was complete the day it was compiled; however, new studies are frequently published on this important medicinal plant. Visit www.pubmed.gov to access the latest studies cataloged at the U.S. National Library of Medicine (PubMed). More information and periodic updated references on the research on chanca piedra can be found in the Rain-Tree Tropical Plant Database file online at www.rain-tree.com/chanca.htm.

Chapter 1. What Is Chanca Piedra?

Ankuret, R., et al. "*Phyllanthus amarus*: an ample therapeutic potential herb." *Int. J. Res. Ayurv. Pharm.* 2011; 2(4): 1096–1099.

Bagalkotkar, G., et al. "Phytochemicals from *Phyllanthus niruri* Linn. and their pharmacological properties: A review." *J. Pharm. Pharmacol.* 2006 Dec; 58(12): 1559–70.

Calixto, J., "A review of the genus *Phyllanthus*: their chemistry, pharmacology, and therapeutic potential." 1998; *Med. Res. Rev.* 18: 225–258.

Islam, A., et al. "Phytopharmacology of *Phyllanthus amarus*: an overview." *Pharmacology.* 2008; 3: 202–209.

Joseph, B., et al. "An overview: pharmacognostic properties of *Phyllanthus amarus* Linn" *Int. J. Pharmacol.* 2011; 7(1): 40–45.

Kamruzzamn, H., et al. "A review on ethnomedicinal, phytochemical and pharmacological properties of *Phyllanthus niruri.*" *J. Med. Plant. Stud.* 2016; 4(6): 173–180.

Kaur, N., et al. "Phytochemistry and pharmacology of *Phyllanthus niruri* L.: A review." *Phytother. Res.* 2017 July; (31)7: 980–1004.

Lee, N., et al. "The pharmacological potential of *Phyllanthus niruri.*" *J. Pharma. Phamacol.* 2016 Mar; 68: 953–969.

Mao, X., et al. "The genus *Phyllanthus*: An ethnopharmacological, phytochemical, and pharmacological review." *Evid. Based Complement. Altern.* 2016; 2016: 1–36.

Narendra, K., et al. "*Phyllanthus niruri*: a review on its ethnobotanical, phytochemical and pharmacological profile." *J. Pharma. Res.* 2012; 5(9): 4681–4691.

Patel, J., et al. "*Phyllanthus amarus*: ethnomedicinal uses, phytochemistry and pharmacology: a review." *J. Ethnopharmacol.* 2011 Nov; 138(2): 286–313.

Chapter 2 The Power of Polyphenols

Anhe, F., et al. "Polyphenols and type 2 diabetes: A prospective review." *Pharma. Nutrition.* 2013; 1: 105–114.

Aruoma, O., et al. "Nutrition and health aspects of free radicals and antioxidants." *Food Chem. Toxicol.* 1994; 32: 671–83.

Ashok, B., et al. "The aging paradox: Free radical theory of aging." *Exp. Gerontol.* 1999; 34: 293–303.

Assini, E., et al. "Antiobesity effects of anthocyanins in preclinical and clinical studies." *Oxid. Med. Cell. Longev.* 2017; 2017: 2740364.

Bagchi, K., and Puri, S. "Free radicals and antioxidants in health and disease." *East Mediterranean Health J.* 1998; 4: 350–60.

Bijak, M., et al. "Popular naturally occurring antioxidants as potential anticoagulant drugs." *Chem. Biol. Interact.* 2016 Sep; 257: 35–45.

Callejo, M., et al. "Impact of nutrition on pulmonary arterial hypertension." *Nutrients.* 2020 Jan; 12(1): E169.

Cheeseman, K., et al. "An introduction to free radical biochemistry." *Br. Med. Bull.* 1993 Jul; 49(3): 481–93.

Chen, Y., et al. "Polyphenols and oxidative stress in atherosclerosis-related ischemic heart disease and stroke." *Oxid. Med. Cell. Longev.* 2017; 2017: 8526438.

Correa, T., et al. "The two-way polyphenols-microbiota interactions and their effects on obesity and related metabolic diseases." *Front. Nutr.* 2019 Dec; 6: 188.

Davinelli, S., et al. "Cytoprotective polyphenols against chronological skin aging and cutaneous photodamage." *Curr. Pharm. Des.* 2018; 24(2): 99–105.

Dilberger, B., et al. "Polyphenols and metabolites enhance survival in rodents and nematodes-impact of mitochondria." *Nutrients.* 2019 Aug; 11(8): E1886.

Dryden, G., et al. "Polyphenols and gastrointestinal diseases." *Curr. Opin. Gastroenterol.* 2006 Mar; 22(2): 165–170.

Grosso, G., et al. "Dietary polyphenol intake and risk of type 2 diabetes in the Polish arm of the health, alcohol and psychosocial factors in eastern Europe (HAPIEE) study." *Br. J. Nutr.* 2017 Jul 14; 118(1): 60–68.

Gupta, R., et al. "Oxidative stress and antioxidants in disease and cancer: a review." *Asian Pac. J. Cancer Prev.* 2014; 15: 4405–4409.

He, L., et al. "Antioxidants maintain cellular redox homeostasis by elimination of reactive oxygen species." *Cell. Physiol. Biochem.* 2017; 44: 532–553.

Hua, J., et al. "Dietary polyphenols turn fat "brown": A narrative review of the possible mechanisms." *Trends Food Sci. Technol.* 2020 Mar; 97: 221–232.

Hussain, T., et al. "Oxidative stress and inflammation: what polyphenols can do for us? *Oxid. Med. Cell. Longev.* 2016; 2016: 7432797.

Karim, N., et al. "An increasing role of polyphenols as novel therapeutics for Alzheimer's: A review." *Med. Chem.* 2019; Nov 5. (ahead of print)

Kim, Y., et al. "Polyphenols and glycemic control." *Nutrients.* 2016 Jan; 8(1): 17.

Li, A., et al. "Resources and biological activities of natural polyphenols." *Nutrients.* 2014 Dec; 6(12): 6020–6047.

Liu, J., et al. "Beneficial effects of dietary polyphenols on high-fat diet-induced obesity linking with modulation of gut microbiota." *J. Agric. Food Chem.* 2020 Jan; 68(1): 33–47.

Lobo, V., et al. "Free radicals, antioxidants and functional foods: Impact on human health." *Pharmacogn. Rev.* 2010 Jul-Dec; 4(8): 118–126.

Majidinia, M., et al. "Targeting miRNAs by polyphenols: Novel therapeutic strategy for aging." *Biochem. Pharmacol.* 2020 Mar; 173: 113688.

Marchesi, J., et al. "The gut microbiota and host health: a new clinical frontier." *Gut.* 2016 Feb; 65(2): 330–9.

Marin, L., et al. "Bioavailability of dietary polyphenols and gut microbiota metabolism: antimicrobial properties." *Biomed. Res. Int.* 2015; 2015: 905215.

Matsuda, M., et al. "Increased oxidative stress in obesity: implications for metabolic syndrome, diabetes, hypertension, dyslipidemia, atherosclerosis, and cancer." *Obes. Res. Clin. Pract.* 2013; 7: e330–e341.

Niedzwiecki, A., et al. "Anticancer efficacy of polyphenols and their combinations." *Nutrients.* 2016 Sep; 8(9): 552.

Pacheco-Ordaz, R., et al. "Effect of phenolic compounds on the growth of selected probiotic and pathogenic bacteria." *Lett. Appl. Microbiol.* 2018 Jan; 66(1): 25–31.

Pham-Huv, L., et al. "Free radicals, antioxidants in disease and health." *Int. J. Biomed. Sci.* 2008 Jun; 4(2): 89–96.

Poti, F., et al. "Polyphenol health effects on cardiovascular and neurodegenerative disorders: a review and meta-analysis." *Int. J. Mol. Sci.* 2019 Jan; 20(2): 351.

Rienks, J., et al. "Association of polyphenol biomarkers with cardiovascular disease and mortality risk: A systematic review and meta-analysis of observational studies." *Nutrients.* 2017 Apr; 9(4): 415.

Rock, C., "Update on biological characteristics of the antioxidant micronutrients - Vitamin C, Vitamin E and the carotenoids." *J. Am. Diet. Assoc.* 1996; 96: 693–702.

Rowland, I., et al. "Gut microbiota functions: metabolism of nutrients and other food components." *Eur. J. Nutr.* 2018 Feb; 57(1): 1–24.

Russo, G., et al. "Mechanisms of aging and potential role of selected polyphenols in extending healthspan." *Biochem. Pharmacol.* 2019 Nov 21: 113719.

Sagnoun, Z., et al. "Free radicals and antioxidants: human physiology, pathology and therapeutic aspects." *Therapie.* 1997 Jul–Aug; 52(4): 251–70.

Silva, R., et al. "Polyphenols from food and natural products: neuroprotection and safety." *Antioxidants.* 2020 Jan; 9(1): E61.

Tangney, C., et al. "Polyphenols, inflammation, and cardiovascular disease." *Curr. Atheroscler. Rep.* 2013 May; 15(5): 324.

Valko, M., et al. "Free radicals and antioxidants in normal physiological functions and human disease." *Review. Int. J. Biochem. Cell Biol.* 2007; 39: 44–84.

Xu, D., et al. "Natural antioxidants in foods and medicinal plants: extraction, assessment and resources." *Int. J. Mol. Sci.* 2017 Jan; 18(1): 96.

Young, I. and Woodside, J. "Antioxidants in health and disease." *J. Clin. Pathol.* 2001; 54: 176–186.

Zang, H., et al. "Dietary polyphenols, oxidative stress and antioxidant and anti-inflammatory effects." *Curr. Opin. Food Sci.* 216 Apr; 8: 33–42.

Zhou, Y., et al. "Natural polyphenols for prevention and treatment of cancer." *Nutrients.* 2016 Aug; 8(8): 515.

Polyphenols in Chanca Piedra

Azam, M., et al. "Phyllanthin: a potential lead molecule for the future." *Int. J. Pharmacog. Phytochem. Res.* 2017; 9(8); 1081–1089.

Bagalkotkar, G., et al. "Phytochemicals from *Phyllanthus niruri* Linn. and their pharmacological properties: a review." *J. Pharma. Pharmacol.* 2006; 58: 1559–1570.

Elfahmi, et al. "Lignans from cell suspension cultures of *Phyllanthus niruri*, an Indonesian medicinal plant." *J. Nat. Prod.* 2006; 69: 55–58.

Huang, R., et al. "Screening of 25 compounds isolated from *Phyllanthus* species for anti-human hepatitis B virus *in vitro*." *Phytother. Res.* 2003; 17: 449–453.

Hukeri, V., et al. "Hypoglycemic activity of flavonoids of *Phyllanthus* in rats." *Fitoterapia.* 1988; 59: 68–70.

Ishimaru, K., et al. "Phenolic constituents in tissue cultures of *Phyllanthus niruri*." *Phytochemistry.* 1992; 31: 2015–2018.

Kamruzzamn, H., et al. "A review on ethnomedicinal, phytochemical and pharmacological properties of *Phyllanthus niruri*." *J. Med. Plant. Stud.* 2016; 4(6): 173–180.

Kassuya, C., et al. "Anti-inflammatory properties of extracts, fractions and lignans isolated from *Phyllanthus amarus*." *Planta Med.* 2005 71: 721–726.

Kaur, N., et al. "Phytochemistry and pharmacology of *Phyllanthus niruri* L.: A review." *Phytother. Res.* 2017 July; (31)7: 980–1004.

Kumar, S., et al. "Identification and characterization of phenolics and terpenoids from ethanolic extracts of *Phyllanthus* species by HPLC-ESI-QTOF-MS/MS." *J. Pharm. Anal.* 2017; 7: 214–222.

Li., X., et al. "Chemical component and bioactivities of *Phyllanthus niruri* L." *Tianran Chanwu Yanjiu Yu Kaifa.* 2007; 19(5): 890–896.

Londhe, J., et al. "Antioxidant activity of some polyphenol constituents of the medicinal plant *Phyllanthus amarus* Linn." *Redox Report.* 2008; 13(5): 199–207.

Ramandeep, K., et al. "Phytochemical screening of *Phyllanthus niruri* collected from Kerala region and its antioxidant and antimicrobial potentials." *J. Pharm. Sci. Res.* 2017; 9: 1312–1316.

Than, N., et al. "Niruriflavone, a new antioxidant flavone sulfonic acid from *Phyllanthus niruri*." *Z. Naturforsch.* 2006; 61b: 57–60.

Chapter 3. Chanca Piedra's Actions on the Kidneys

Adejuwon, A., et al. "Protective effect of the aqueous leaf and seed extract of *Phyllanthus amarus* on gentamicin and acetaminophen-induced nephrotoxic rats." *J. Ethnopharmacol.* 2008; 118: 318–323.

Adjene, J., et al. "Histological effects of chronic administration of *Phyllanthus amarus* on the kidney of adult Wistar rat." *N. Am. J. Med. Sci.* 2010 Apr; 2(4): 193–5.

Agarwal, K., et al. "Investigating antiuroliathiatic potential of *Phyllanthus niruri* L. a member of the family Euphorbiaceae." *Am. J. Phytomed. Clinic. Ther.* 2014: 2(7): 423–431.

Ahmed, S., et al. "*In vitro* urolithiasis models: An evaluation of prophylactic management against kidney stones." *J. Pharmacog. Phytochem.* 2016; 5(3): 28–35.

Barros, M., et al. "Effect of extract of *Phyllanthus niruri* on crystal deposition in experimental urolithiasis." *Urol. Res.* 2006 Dec; 34(6): 351–7.

Barros, M., et al. "Effects of an aqueous extract from *Phyllanthus niruri* on calcium oxalate crystallization *in vitro*." *Urol. Res.* 2003; 30(6): 374–9.

Boeira, V., et al. "Effects of the hydroalcoholic extract of *Phyllanthus niruri* and its isolated compounds on cyclophosphamide-induced hemorrhagic cystitis in mouse." *Naunyn. Schmiedebergs. Arch. Pharmacol.* 2011 Sep; 384(3): 265–75.

References

Boim, M., et al. "*Phyllanthus niruri* as a promising alternative treatment for nephrolithiasis." *Int. Braz. J. Urol.* 2010 Nov–Dec; 36(6): 657–64.

Calixto, J., et al. "Antispasmodic effects of an alkaloid extracted from *Phyllanthus sellowianus*: a comparative study with papaverine." *Braz. J. Med. Biol. Res.* 1984; 17: 313–321.

Campos, A., et al. "*Phyllanthus niruri* inhibits calcium oxalate endocytosis by renal tubular cells: its role in urolithiasis." *Nephron.* 1999; 81(4): 393–97.

Cealan, A., et al. "Evaluation of the efficacy of *Phyllanthus niruri* standardized extract combined with magnesium and vitamin B6 for the treatment of patients with uncomplicated nephrolithiasis." *Med. Pharm. Rep.* 2019 Apr; 92(2): 153–157.

Celia, A., et al. "May *Phyllanthus niruri* (Uriston®) affect the efficacy of ESWL on renal stones? A prospective, randomised short term study." *J. Urology.* 2005 Apr; 173(4S): 460.

Cos, P., et al. "Structure-activity relationship and classification of flavonoids as inhibitors of xanthine oxidase and superoxide scavengers." *J. Nat. Prod.* 1998; 61: 71–6.

de Oliveira, V., et al. "Aspects of current use of *Phyllanthus niruri* (break-stone) in the treatment of kidney lithiasis." *REAS/EJCH.* 2019; 11(15): e1386.

Escribano, J., et al. "Dietary interventions for preventing complications in idiopathic hypercalciuria." *Cochrane Database Syst. Rev.* 2014 Feb; (2): CD006022.

Ettinger, B., et al. "Potassium-magnesium citrate is an effective prophylaxis against recurrent calcium oxalate nephrolithiasis." *J. Urol.* 1997; 158: 2069–2073.

Eweka, A., et al. "Effects of oral administration of *Phyllanthus amarus* leaf extract on the kidneys of adult Wistar rats: a histological study." *Afr. J. Tradit. Complement. Altern. Med.* 2011; 8(3): 307–11.

Freitas, A., et al. "The effect of *Phyllanthus niruri* on urinary inhibitors of calcium oxalate crystallization and other factors associated with renal stone formation." *B. J. U. Int.* 2002; 89(9): 829–34.

Giribabu, N., et al. "Aqueous extract of *Phyllanthus niruri* leaves displays *in vitro* antioxidant activity and prevents the elevation of oxidative stress in the kidney of streptozotocin-induced diabetic male rats." *Evid. Based Complement. Alternat. Med.* 2014; 2014: 834815.

Giribabu, N., et al. "*Phyllanthus niruri* leaves aqueous extract improves kidney functions, ameliorates kidney oxidative stress, inflammation, fibrosis and apoptosis and enhances kidney cell proliferation in adult male rats with Diabetes mellitus." *J. Ethnopharmacol.* 2017 Jun 9; 205: 123–137.

Hatano, T., et al. "Effects of interaction of tannins with co-existing substances. VII. Inhibitory effects of tannins and related polyphenols on xanthine oxidase." *Chem. Pharm. Bull.* 1990; 38: 1224–9.

Kasote, D., et al. "Herbal remedies for urinary stones used in India and China: A review." *J. Ethnopharmacol.* 2017 May; 203: 55–68.

Khare, P., et al. "Study on *in vitro* anti-lithiatic activity of *Phyllanthus niruri* Linn. leaves by homogenous precipitation and turbiditory method." *Int. J. Pharm. Pharmaceut. Sci.* 2014; 6(4): 124–127.

Kieley, S., et al. "Ayurvedic medicine and renal calculi." *J. Endourol.* 2008; 22(8): 1613–6.

Kitisin, T., et al. "Pharmacological studies. *Phyllanthus niruri.*" *Sirriaj. Hosp. Gaz.* 1952; 4: 641–649.

Mans, D., et al. "Assessment of eight popularly used plant-derived preparations for their spasmolytic potential using the isolated guinea pig ileum." *Pharma. Bio.* 2004; 42: 422–429.

Marques, L. "*Phyllanthus niruri* (stone breaker) in the treatment of urolithiasis: Proposed documentation for simplified registration as a herbal medicine." *Revista Fitos.* 2010 Sep; 5(3): 20–33.

Micali, S., et al. "Can *Phyllanthus niruri* affect the efficacy of extracorporeal shock wave lithotripsy for renal stones? A randomized, prospective, long-term study." *J. Urol.* 2006 Sep; 176(3): 1020–2.

Murugaiyah V, et al. "Antihyperuricemic lignans from the leaves of *Phyllanthus niruri.*" *Planta Med.* 2006 Nov; 72(14): 1262–7.

Murugaiyah, V., et al. "Mechanisms of antihyperuricemic effect of *Phyllanthus niruri* and its lignan constituents." *J. Ethnopharmacol.* 2009 Jul; 124(2): 233–9.

Nishiura, J., et al. "*Phyllanthus niruri* normalizes elevated urinary calcium levels in calcium stone forming (CSF) patients." *Urol. Res.* 2004 Oct; 32(5): 362–6.

Priya, A. and Sudha, V. "Anti-urolithiatic activity of medicinal plants and Siddha formulatory medicine – A review." *J. Res. Biosci. Sci.* 2020 Jan–Mar; 3(1): 7–12.

Pucci, N., et al. "Effect of *Phyllanthus niruri* on metabolic parameters of patients with kidney stone: a perspective for disease prevention." *Int. Braz. J. Urol.* 2018 Jul–Aug; 44(4): 758–764.

Ramsout, R., et al. "Investigation of the effects of *Phyllanthus niruri* L. on *in vitro* calcium oxalate crystallization." *Eur. Urol. Suppl.* 2011; 10: 461–474.

Rapa, S., et al. "Inflammation and oxidative stress in chronic kidney disease—potential therapeutic role of minerals, vitamins and plant-derived metabolites." *Int. J. Mol. Sci.* 2020; 21: 263.

Reungjui, S., et al. "Magnesium status of patients with renal stones and its effect on urinary citrate excretion." *B.J.U. Int.* 2002 Nov; 90(7): 635–9.

Rodgers, A., et al. "Herbal preparations affect the kinetic factors of calcium oxalate crystallization in synthetic urine: implications for kidney stone therapy." *Urolithiasis*. 2014 Jun; 42(3): 221–5.

Santos, D. "Natural Products in the Treatment of Nephrolithiasis" In: Schor, N. (ed.), *Renal Calculosis: Pathophysiology, Diagnosis and Treatment*. São Paulo, Brasil. Ed. Sarvier. 1995; pp. 221–5.

Schuler, T., et al. "Medical expulsive therapy as an adjunct to improve shock-wave lithotripsy outcomes: a systematic review and meta-analysis." *J. Endourol.* 2009; 23(3): 387–93.

Woottisin, S., et al. "Effects of *Orthosiphon grandiflorus, Hibiscus sabdariffa* and *Phyllanthus amarus* extracts on risk factors for urinary calcium oxalate stones in rats." *J. Urol.* 2011 Jan; 185(1): 323–8.

Wright, C., et al. "Herbal medicines as diuretics: a review of the scientific evidence." *J. Ethnopharmacol.* 2007 Oct; 114(1): 1–31.

Yao, A. et al. "The acute diuretic effect of an ethanolic fraction of *Phyllanthus amarus* (Euphorbiaceae) in rats involves prostaglandins." *BMC Complement. Altern. Med.* 2018 Mar; 18(1): 94.

Chapter 4. Chanca Piedra and Emerging Infectious Diseases

Antibacterial & Antifungal Actions

Agrawal, A., et al. "Evaluation of inhibitory effect of the plant *Phyllanthus amarus* against dermatophytic fungi *Microsporum gypseum*." *Biomed. Environ. Sci.* 2004 Sep; 17(3): 359–65.

Ahamath, J., et al. "Phytochemical screening and antimicrobial activity of *Phyllanthus niruri*." *J. Adv. Appl. Sci. Res.* 2017; 1: 7.

Ajibade, V., et al. "Antibacterial activity of saponin and alkaloidal extracts of whole plant of *Phyllanthus niruri* L. (Syn. *P. franternus* Webster)." *Pak. J. Sci. Ind. Res. Ser. B: Biol. Sci.* 2011; 5 (1): 47–52.

Ajibade, V., et al. "Antibacterial activity of saponin extracted from *Phyllanthus niruri* on methicillin-resistant *Staphylococcus aureus* (MRSA)." *J. Complement. Alt. Med. Res.* 2019; 7(1): 1–9.

Akinjogunia, O., et al. "Antibacterial activity of ethanolic extracts of *Phyllanthus amarus* against extended spectrum ß-lactamase producing *Escherichia coli* isolated from stool samples of HIV sero-positive patients with or without diarrhoea." *Afr. J. Pharm. Pharmacol.* 2010; 4(6): 402–407.

Amin, Z., et al. "Assessment of *in vitro* antioxidant, antibacterial and immune activation potentials of aqueous and ethanol extracts of *Phyllanthus niruri*." *J. Sci. Food Agric.* 2012 Jul; 92(9): 1874–7.

Bhat, S., et al. "Preclinical screening of *Phyllanthus amarus* ethanolic extract for its analgesic and antimicrobial activity." *Pharmacognosy Res.* 2014 Oct–Dec; 7(4): 378–84.

Boakye, Y., et al. "Anti-infective properties and time-kill kinetics of *Phyllanthus muellerianus* and its major constituent, geraniin." *Med. Chem.* 2016; 6: 95–104.

Ekwenye, U., et al. "Antibacterial effect of *Phyllanthus niruri* (Chanca Piedra) on three enteropathogens in man." *Intl. J. Mol. Adv. Sci.* 2006; 2(2): 184–189.

Farouk, A., et al. "Antimicrobial activity of certain Sudanese; plants used in folkloric medicine. Screening for antibacterial activity (I)." *Fitoterapia* 1983; 54(1): 3–7.

Gbadamosi, I., et al. "Antibacterial attributes of extracts of *Phyllantus amarus* and *Phyllanthus niruri* on *Escherichia coli* the causal organism of urinary tract infection." *J. Pharm. Phytother.* 2015 May; 7(5): 80–86.

Gunawan, I., et al. "Isolation, characterization and antibacterial activity of triterpenoid compounds fraction chloroform bark *Phyllanthus niruri* L." *World Pharm. Pharm. Sci.* 2016; 5: 357–364.

Hidanah, S., et al. "Effects of meniran (*Phyllanthus niruri* L.) administration on leukocyte profile of broiler chickens infected with *Mycoplasma gallisepticum*." *Vet. World.* 2018 Jun; (6): 834–839.

Hoffman, B., et al. "Screening of antibacterial and antifungal activities of ten medicinal plants from Ghana." *Pharma. Bio.* 2004; 42(1): 13–17.

Ibrahim, D., et al. "Antimicrobial activity of crude methanolic extract from *Phyllanthus niruri*." *Nat. Prod. Comm.* 2013; 8(4): 493–496.

Kanthimathi, M., et al. "Antibacterial effects of *Emblica officinalis* and *Phyllanthus niruri* crude extracts against bacterial pathogens." *Intl. J. Pharm. Clin. Sci.* 2013 Jun; 3(3): 20–23.

Kaur, R., et al. "Phytochemical screening of *Phyllanthus niruri* collected from Kerala region and its antioxidant and antimicrobial potentials." *J. Pharm. Sci. Res.* 2017; 9(8): 1312–1316.

Kaur, B., et al. "Evaluation of anti-*Helicobacter pylori* (DSMZ 10242) activity and qualitative analysis of quercetin by HPLC in *Phyllanthus niruri* Linn." *World J. Pharm. Pharm.* Sci. 2016: 5: 1691–1706.

Kloucek, P., et al. "Antibacterial screening of some Peruvian medicinal plants used in Calleria District." *J. Ethnopharmacol.* 2005 Jun; 99(2): 309–12.

Legba, B., et al. "Evaluation of *in-vivo* anti-Salmonella activity of *Uvaria chamae, Lantana camara* and *Phyllantus amarus* used in Benin, West Africa." *BMC Vet. Res.* 2020 Feb; 16(1): 49.

Legba, B., et al. "Toxicological characterization of six plants of the Beninese pharmacopoeia used in the treatment of salmonellosis." *J. Toxicol.* 2019 Jul; 2019: 3530659.

Lopez, C., et al. "Antimicrobial activity of medicinal plant extracts against foodborne spoilage and pathogenic microorganisms." *J. Kas. Nat. Sci.* 2003; 37: 460–467.

Ma'at, S. "Antimycotic and immunomodulator in mycosis: *Phyllanthus niruri* extract as a natural immunomodulator." Paper presented at the periodic scientific meeting of the Association of Human and Animal Mycological Medicine, Solo. Central Java, September 2001.

Mazumder, A., et al. "Antimicrobial potentiality of *Phyllanthus amarus* against drug resistant pathogens." *Nat. Prod. Res.* 2006; 20(4): 323–6.

Mondal, R., et al. "Antimicrobial activity of natural products from medicinal plants." *J. Agroeco. Nat. Resour.* 2018 Mar; 5(1): 63–69.

Narayanan, A., et al. "Antibacterial activity of selected medicinal plants against multiple antibiotic resistant uropathogens: a study from Kolli Hills, Tamil Nadu, India." *Benef. Microbes.* 2011 Sep; 2(3): 235–43.

Obiagwu, I., et al. "Studies on antibacterial effect of the leaves of *Phyllanthus niruri* on some enteric pathogens." *Nig. J. Biotech.* 2011; 23: 22–27.

Okigbo, R., et al. "Antimicrobial effects of *Piper guineense* 'Uziza' and *Phyllanthus amarus* 'Ebe-benizo' on *Candida albicans* and *Streptococcus faecalis*." *Acta Microbiol. Immunol. Hung.* 2007 Dec; 54(4): 353–66.

Oluboyo, B., et al. "Inhibitory effects of *Phyllanthus amarus* extracts on the growth of some pathogenic microorganisms." *Afr. J. Clin. Exp. Microbiol.* 2016; 17: 166–172.

Rani, J., et al. "Antibacterial properties of extracts of Indian medicinal plants: *Syzygium alternifolium, Phyllanthus niruri* and *Rubia cordifolia*." *Biomed. Pharmacol. J.* 2010; 3(1): 123–128.

Ranilla, L, et al. "Antimicrobial activity of an Amazon medicinal plant (Chanca piedra) (*Phyllanthus niruri* L.) against *Helicobacter pylori* and lactic acid bacteria." *Phytother. Res.* 2012 Jun; 26(6): 791–9.

Ribeiro, A., et al. "Antimicrobial activity of *Phyllanthus amarus* Schumach. & Thonn and inhibition of the NorA efflux pump of *Staphylococcus aureus* by phyllanthin." *Microb. Pathog.* 2019 May; 130: 242–246.

Senjobi, C., et al. "Antibacterial and antifungal activities of leaf extracts of *Phyllanthus amarus* Schum and Thonn." *J. Pharmacogn. Phytother.* 2017; 9: 6–10.

Shanmugam, B., et al. "Antibacterial activity and phytochemical screening of *Phyllanthus niruri* in ethanolic, methanolic and aqueous extracts." *Int. J. Pharm. Sci. Rev. Res.* 2014 Jul–Aug; 27(2): 85–89.

Sharadadevi, D., et al. "*In vitro* antimicrobial synergism of three Indian medicinal plant extracts alone and in combination with different antimicrobials against pathogenic bacterial strains." *Int. Res. J. Pharm.* 2019 Jan; 10 (3): 120–126.

Sunitha, J., et al. "Antimicrobial effect of leaves of *Phyllanthus niruri* and *Solanum nigrum* on caries causing bacteria: an *in vitro* study." *J. Clin. Diagn. Res.* 2017 Jun; 11(6): KC01–KC04.

Uzor, B., et al. "Phytochemical composition and antimicrobial potential of *Phyllanthus amarus* leaf extract against some clinical isolates." *Niger. J. Microbiol.* 2016; 30: 3464–3467.

Valle, D., et al. "Antibacterial activities of ethanol extracts of Philippine medicinal plants against multidrug-resistant bacteria." *Asian Pac. J. Trop. Biomed* 2015; 5(7): 532–540.

Anti-Malarial and Anti-Parasitic Actions

Ajala, T., et al. "The antiplasmodial effect of the extracts and formulated capsules of *Phyllanthus amarus* on *Plasmodium yoelii* infection in mice." *Asian Pac. J. Trop. Med.* 2011 Apr; 4(4): 283–7.

Appiah-Opong, R., et al. "Antiplasmodial activity of extracts of *Tridax procumbens* and *Phyllanthus amarus* in *in vitro Plasmodium falciparum* culture systems." *Ghana Med. J.* 2011 Dec; 45(4): 143–50.

Chowdhury, S., et al. "The lignan niranthin poisons *Leishmania donovani* topoisomerase IB and favours a Th1 immune response in mice." *EMBO Mol. Med.* 2012 Oct; 4(10): 1126–43.

Cimanga, R., et al. "*In vitro* antiplasmodial activity of callus culture extracts and fractions from fresh apical stems of *Phyllanthus niruri* L. (Euphorbiaceae): part 2." *J. Ethnopharmacol.* 2004 Dec; 95(2-3): 399–404.

Dapper, D., et al. "Antiplasmodial effects of the aqueous extract of *Phyllantus amarus* Schumach and Thonn against *Plasmodium berghei* in Swiss albino mice." *Niger. J. Physiol. Sci.* 2007 Jun–Dec; 22(1-2): 19–25.

de Oliveira, C., et al. "*Schistosoma mansoni*: *In vivo* evaluation of *Phyllanthus amarus* hexanic and ethanolic extracts." *Exp. Parasitol.* 2017 Dec; 183: 56–63.

Fasinu, P., et al. "Modulation of Cytochrome P450, P-glycoprotein and Pregnane X Receptor by selected antimalarial herbs-implication for herb-drug interaction." *Molecules.* 2017 Nov; 22(12): E2049.

Haslinda, M., et al. "*In vitro* antiplasmodial activity, macronutrients and trace metals in the medicinal plants: *Phyllanthus spp.* and *Alpinia conchigera* Griff." *Trop. Biomed.* 2015 Mar; 32(1): 129–39.

Ifeoma, O., et al. "Isolation, fractionation and evaluation of the antiplasmodial properties of *Phyllanthus niruri* resident in its chloroform fraction." *Asian Pac. J. Trop. Med.* 2013 Mar; 6(3): 169–75.

Kabiru, A., et al. "Evaluation of haematological changes in *Plasmodium-berghei*-infected mice administered with aqueous extract *of Phyllanthus amarus.*" *Pak. J. Biol. Sci.* 2013 Jun; 16(11): 510–6.

Kamaraj, C., et al. "Antimalarial activities of medicinal plants traditionally used in the villages of Dharmapuri regions of South India." *J. Ethnopharmacol.* 2012 Jun 14; 141(3): 796–802.

Keluskar, P., et al. "Ethnopharmacology guided screening of traditional Indian herbs for selective inhibition of *Plasmodium* specific lactate dehydrogenase." *J. Ethnopharmacol.* 2012 Oct; 144(1): 201–7.

Komlaga, G., et al. "Antiplasmodial securinega alkaloids from *Phyllanthus fraternus*: Discovery of natural(+)-allonorsecurinine." *Tetrahedron Lett.* 2017; 58: 3754–3756.

Kolodziej, H., et al. "Tannins and related compounds induce nitric oxide synthase and cytokines gene expressions in *Leishmania major*-infected macrophage-like RAW 264.7 cells." *Bioorg. Med. Chem.* 2005 Dec; 13(23): 6470–6.

Mesia, L., et al. "*In-vitro* antimalarial activity of *Cassia occidentalis, Morinda morindoides* and *Phyllanthus niruri.*" *Ann. Trop. Med. Parasitol.* 2001; 95(1): 47–57.

Mustofa, S., et al. "*In vitro* and *in vivo* antiplasmodial activity and cytotoxicity of extracts of *Phyllanthus niruri* L. herbs traditionally used to treat malaria in Indonesia." *Southeast Asian J. Trop. Med. Public Health.* 2007 Jul; 38(4): 609–15.

Ndjonka, D., et al. "*In vitro* activity of extracts and isolated polyphenols from West African medicinal plants against *Plasmodium falciparum.*" *Parasitol. Res.* 2012 ;111(2): 827–834.

Ojezele, M., et al. "Impact of generic antimalarial or *Phyllanthus amarus* and vitamin co-administration on antioxidant status of experimental mice infested with *Plasmodium berghei.*" *Beni-Suef Univ. J. Basic Appl. Sci.* 2017; 6: 260–265.

Rahuman, A., et al. "Larvicidal activity of some Euphorbiaceae plant extracts against *Aedes aegypti* and *Culex quinquefasciatus* (Diptera: Culicidae)." *Parasitol. Res.* 2008 Apr; 102(5): 867–73.

Shakil, N., et al. "Nematicidal prenylated flavanones from *Phyllanthus niruri.*" *Phytochemistry.* 2008 Feb; 69(3): 759–64.

Subeki, S., et al. "Anti-babesial and anti-plasmodial compounds from *Phyllanthus niruri.*" *J. Nat. Prod.* 2005; 68(4): 537–9.

Tona, L., et al. "Antimalarial activity of 20 crude extracts from nine African medicinal plants used in Kinshasa, Congo." *J. Ethnopharmacol.* 1999; 68(1/3): 193–203.

Tona, L., et al. "*In vitro* antiplasmodial activity of extracts and fractions from seven medicinal plants used in the Democratic Republic of Congo." *J. Ethnopharmacol.* 2004 Jul; 93(1): 27–32.

Traore, M., et al. "*In vitro* and *in vivo* antiplasmodial activity of 'saye', an herbal remedy used in Burkina Faso traditional medicine." *Phytother. Res.* 2008; 22(4): 550–1.

Venkatesalu, V., et al. "*In vitro* anti-plasmodial activity of some traditionally used medicinal plants against *Plasmodium falciparum.*" *Parasitol. Res.* 2012 Jul; 111(1): 497–501.

Yerbanga, R. et al. "Antimalarial plant remedies from Burkina Faso: their potential for prophylactic use." *J. Ethnopharmacol.* 2012 Mar; 140(2): 255–60.

Antiviral Actions

Bagalkotkar, G., et al. "Phytochemicals from *Phyllanthus niruri* Linn. and their pharmacological properties: a review." *J. Pharm. Pharmacol.* 2006 Dec; 58(12): 1559–70.

Baiguera, C., et al. "*Phyllanthus niruri* versus placebo for chronic hepatitis B virus infection: A randomized controlled trial." *Complement Med. Res.* 2018; 25(6): 376–382.

Blumberg, B., et al. "Hepatitis B virus and hepatocellular carcinoma—treatment of HBV carriers with *Phyllanthus amarus.*" *Cancer Detect. Prev.* 1989; 14: 195–201.

Cheng, H., et al. "Excoecarianin, isolated from *Phyllanthus urinaria* Linnea, inhibits *Herpes simplex* virus type 2 infection through inactivation of viral particles." *Evid. Based Complement. Alternat. Med.* 2011; 2011: 259103.

Cheng, Y., et al. "Clinical study of *Phyllanthus* pill on treating chronic hepatitis B." *Zhongxiyi Jiehe. Ganbing. Zazhi.* 2009; 19(17): 195–197.

Chitra, R., et al. "Estimation of anti-hepatic viral compounds in *Phyllanthus amarus in vitro* cultures." *J. Hortic. Sci.* 2016; 3: 62–65.

Cui, Q., et al. "Lignans and their derivatives from plants as antivirals." *Molecules* 2020 Jan; 25(1): 183.

Dinesh, S., et al. "Molecular docking and simulation studies of *Phyllanthus amarus* phytocompounds against structural and nucleocapsid proteins of white spot syndrome virus." *3 Biotech.* 2017; 7: 353.

Dirjomuljono, M., et al. "Symptomatic treatment of acute tonsillo-pharyngitis patients with a combination of *Nigella sativa* and *Phyllanthus niruri* extract." *Int. J. Clin. Pharmacol. Ther.* 2008; 46(6): 295–306.

Faeji, C., et al. "In-ovo biological activities of *Phyllanthus amarus* leaf extracts against Newcastle disease virus." *J. Med. Plants Res.* 2017; 11: 419–425.

Faral-Tello, P., et al. "Cytotoxic, virucidal, and antiviral activity of South American plant and algae extracts." *Sci. World J.* 2012; 2012: 174837.

Huang, R., et al. "Screening of 25 compounds isolated from *Phyllanthus* species for anti-human hepatitis B virus *in vitro.*" *Phytother. Res.* 2003; 17(5): 449–53.

Li, Y., et al. "Anti-hepatitis B viral activity of *Phyllanthus niruri* L (Phyllanthaceae) in HepG2/C3A and SK-HEP-1 cells." *Trop. J. Pharma. Res.* 2017 Aug; 16 (8): 1873–1879.

References

Liu, J., et al. "Genus *Phyllanthus* for chronic Hepatitis B virus infection: A systematic review." *Viral Hepat.* 2001; 8(5): 358–66.

Liu, S., et al. "*In vitro* and *in vivo* anti-hepatitis B virus activities of the lignan niranthin isolated from *Phyllanthus niruri* L." *J. Ethnopharmacol.* 2014 Sep 11; 155(2): 1061–7.

Mohan, M., et al. "Molecular docking studies of phytochemicals from *Phyllanthus niruri* against Hepatitis B DNA Polymerase." *Bioinformation.* 2015 Sep 30; 11(9): 426–31.

Naik, A., et al. "Effects of alkaloidal extract of *Phyllanthus niruri* on HIV replication." *Indian J. Med. Sci.* 2003 Sep; 57(9): 387–93.

Notka, F., et al. "Concerted inhibitory activities of *Phyllanthus amarus* on HIV replication *in vitro* and *ex vivo*." *Antiviral Res.* 2004 Nov; 64(2): 93–102.

Notka, F., et al. "Inhibition of wild-type human immunodeficiency virus and reverse transcriptase inhibitor-resistant variants by *Phyllanthus amarus*." *Antiviral Res.* 2003 Apr; 58(2): 175–186.

Ogata, T., et al. "HIV-1 reverse transcriptase inhibitor from *Phyllanthus niruri*." *AIDS Res. Hum. Retroviruses* 1992; 8(11): 1937–44.

Ott, M., et al. "Use of *Phyllanthus* constituents for treating or preventing infections caused by hepatitis B-viruses." U.S. Patent # US7829124B2. Nov. 2010.

Qi, F., et al. "Traditional Chinese medicine and related active compounds: a review of their role on hepatitis B virus infection." *Drug Discov. Ther.* 2013 Dec; 7(6): 212–24.

Qian-Cutrone, J. "Niruriside, a new HIV REV/RRE binding inhibitor from *Phyllanthus niruri*." *J. Nat. Prod.* 1996; 59(2): 196–99.

Ravikumar, Y., et al. "Inhibition of hepatitis C virus replication by herbal extract: *Phyllanthus amarus* as potent natural source." *Virus Res.* 2011 Jun; 158(1-2): 89–97.

Reddy, B., et al. "A natural small molecule inhibitor corilagin blocks HCV replication and modulates oxidative stress to reduce liver damage." *Antiviral Res.* 2018 Feb; 150: 47–59.

Sarisetyaningtyas, P., et al. "Randomized controlled trial of *Phyllanthus niruri* Linn extract." *Paediatr. Indones.* 2006 Mar–Apr: 46(3-4): 77–81.

Sarma, K., et al. "In silico identification of natural lead molecules from the genus of *Phyllanthus* against hepatitis B virus reverse transcriptase." *Nat. Prod. J.* 2016; 6: 292–304.

Sundaram, D., et al. "Protective efficacy of active compounds from *Phyllanthus amarus* against white spot syndrome virus in freshwater crab (*Paratelphusa hydrodomous*)." Aquac. Res. 2016; 47: 2061–2067.

Thyagarajan, S., et al. "*Phyllanthus amarus* and hepatitis B." *Lancet.* 1990; 336: 949–950.

Thyagarajan, S., et al. "Preliminary study: effect of *Phyllanthus amarus* on chronic carriers of hepatitis B virus." *Lancet.* 1988; 2: 764–766.

Unander, D., et al. "Usage and bioassays in *Phyllanthus* (Euphorbiaceae). IV. Clustering of antiviral uses and other effects." *J. Ethnopharmacol.* 1995; 45: 1–18.

Wang, M., et al. "Herbs of the genus *Phyllanthus* in the treatment of chronic Hepatitis B: Observation with three preparations from different geographic sites." *J. Lab. Clin. Med.* 1995; 126(4): 350–52.

Wei, W., et al. "Lignans with anti-hepatitis B virus activities from *Phyllanthus niruri* L." *Phytother. Res.* 2012 Jul; 26(7): 964–8.

Xin-Hua, W., et al. "A comparative study of *Phyllanthus amarus* compound and interferon in the treatment of chronic viral Hepatitis B." *Southeast Asian J. Trop. Med. Public Health* 2001; 32(1): 140–42.

Yang, C., et al. "The *in vitro* activity of geraniin and 1,3,4,6-tetra-O-galloyl-beta-D-glucose isolated from *Phyllanthus urinaria* against *Herpes simplex* virus type 1 and type 2 infection." *J. Ethnopharmacol.* 2007 Apr; 110(3): 555–8.

Yang, C., et al. "Acetone, ethanol and methanol extracts of *Phyllanthus urinaria* inhibit HSV-2 infection *in vitro.*" *Antiviral Res.* 2005; 67: 24–30.

Immunomodulatory Actions

Amin, Z. "The effect of *Phyllanthus* extract as an additional treatment in tuberculosis patients with minimal and moderately advanced radiological lesion." Dissertation 2005. University of Indonesia, Jakarta.

Bhumyamalaki, et al. "*Phyllanthus niruri* and jaundice in children." *J. Natl. Integ. Med. Ass.* 1983; 25(8): 269–72.

Chowdhury, S., et al. "The lignan niranthin poisons *Leishmania donovani* topoisomerase IB and favours a Th1 immune response in mice." *EMBO Mol. Med.* 2012 Oct; 4(10): 1126–43.

Eze, C., et al. "Immunomodulatory activities of methanol extract of the whole aerial part of *Phyllantus niruri* L." *J. Pharmacogn. Phytother.* 2014; 6: 41–6.

Gambari, R., et al. "Corilagin is a potent inhibitor of NF-κB activity and downregulates TNF-α induced expression of IL-8 gene in cystic fibrosis IB3-1 cells." *Int. Immunopharmacol.* 2012; 13(3): 308–315.

Halim, H., and Saleh, K. "The effectiveness of *Phyllanthus niruri* extract in the management of pulmonary tuberculosis." *Dexa Media* 2005; 18: 103–107.

Ilangkovan, M., et al. "Immunosuppressive effects of the standardized extract of *Phyllanthus amarus* on cellular immune responses in Wistar-Kyoto rats." *Drug Des. Devel. Ther.* 2015 Aug; 9: 4917–30.

Ilangkovan, M., et al. "Inhibitory effects of the standardized extract of

Phyllanthus amarus on cellular and humoral immune responses in Balb/C mice." *Phytother. Res.* 2016 Aug; 30(8): 1330–8.

Ilangkovan, M., et al. "Phyllanthin from *Phyllanthus amarus* inhibits cellular and humoral immune responses in Balb/C mice." *Phytomedicine.* 2016 Nov; 23(12): 1441–1450.

Jantan, I., et al. "An insight into the modulatory effects and mechanisms of action of *Phyllanthus* species and their bioactive metabolites on the immune system." *Front. Pharmacol.* 2019 Aug; 10: 878.

Jatan, I., et al. "Inhibition of chemiluminescence and chemotactic activity of phagocytes *in vitro* by the extracts of selected medicinal plants." *J. Nat. Med.* 2011 Apr; 65(2): 400–5.

Kumar, P., et al. "Effect of *Phyllanthus niruri* extracts on colony forming units of the granulocyte-macrophage series activity in serum of mice." *World J. Pharm. Pharmacol. Sci.* 2015; 4: 1984–92.

Lee, N., et al. "The pharmacological potential of *Phyllanthus niruri*." *J. Pharm. Pharmacol.* 2016; 68: 953–69.

Li, L., et al. "Corilagin interferes with toll-like receptor 3-mediated immune response in Herpes simplex encephalitis." *Front. Mol. Neurosci.* 2019 Apr; 12: 83.

Ma'at, S. "Antimycotic and immunomodulator in mycosis: *Phyllanthus niruri* extract as a natural immunomodulator." Paper presented at the periodic scientific meeting of the Association of Human and Animal Mycological Medicine, Solo. Central Java, September 2001.

Ma'at, S. "*Phyllanthus niruri* L. as an immunostimulator in mice." 1996 Dissertation. University of Airlangga, Surabaya. Indonesia.

Mellinger, C., et al. "Chemical and immunological modifications of an arabinogalactan present in tea preparations of *Phyllanthus niruri* after treatment with gastric fluid." *Int. J. Biol. Macromol.* 2008 Aug; 43(2): 115–20.

Muthulakshmi, M., et al. "Immunostimulatory effect of the aqueous leaf extract of *Phyllanthus niruri* on the specific and nonspecific immune responses of *Oreochromis mossambicus* Peters." *Iran J. Vet. Res.* 2016 Summer; 17(3): 200–202.

Nhu, T., et al. "Plant extract-based diets differently modulate immune responses and resistance to bacterial infection in striped catfish (*Pangasianodon hypophthalmus*)." *Fish Shellfish Immunol.* 2019 Sep; 92: 913–924.

Nhu, T., et al. "Screening of immuno-modulatory potential of different herbal plant extracts using striped catfish (*Pangasianodon hypophthalmus*) leukocyte-based *in vitro* tests." *Fish Shellfish Immunol.* 2019 Oct; 93: 296–307.

Nworu, C., et al. "The effects of *Phyllanthus niruri* aqueous extract on the activation of murine lymphocytes and bone marrow-derived macrophages." *Immunol. Invest.* 2010 Jan; 39(3): 245–67.

Pramayanti, I., et al. "Comparison of success rate of vaginal candidiasis treatment between ketokonazole and combination of ketokonazole-*Phyllanthus niruri* extract." *Dexa Media* 2005; 18: 97–102.

Putri, D., et al. "Immune modulation properties of herbal plant leaves: *Phyllanthus niruri* aqueous extract on immune cells of tuberculosis patient - *in vitro* study." *Nat. Prod. Res.* 2018 Feb; 32(4): 463–467.

Radityawan, D. "The immunomodulatory effect of *Phyllanthus niruri* L on serum IFN-y level in pulmonary tuberculosis patients." *Dexa Media* 2005; 18: 94–96.

Rahfiludin, M., et al. "*Phyllanthus niruri* extract could improve immunoglobulin-M anti phenolic glycolipid-1 level in seropositive contact of Hansen's disease patients." *J. Heath Res.* 2012 Apr; 26(2): 55–77.

Raveinal, R. "The effect of natural immunomodulator (Phyllanti herb extract) administration on cellular immune response of patients with pulmonary tuberculosis." 2003 Thesis. University of Andalas, Padang, Indonesia.

Sarisetyaningtyas, P., et al. "Randomized controlled trial of *Phyllanthus niruri* Linn extract." *Paediatr. Indones.* 2006 Mar–Apr: 46(3-4): 77–81.

Thyagarajan, S. P., et al. "Effect of *Phyllanthus amarus* on chronic carriers of Hepatitis B virus." *Lancet* 1988; 2(8614): 764–66.

Thyagarajan, S., et al. "*In vitro* inactivation of HBsAG by *Eclipta alba* (Hassk.) and *Phyllanthus niruri* (Linn.)." *Indian J. Med. Res.* 1982; 76s: 124–30.

Tjandrawinata, R., et al. "The use of *Phyllanthus niruri* L. as an immunomodulator for the treatment of infectious diseases in clinical settings." *Trop. J. Pharm. Res.* 2017 Aug; 16(8): 1873.

Unander, D., et al. "Usage and bioassays in *Phyllanthus* (Euphorbiaceae). IV. Clustering of antiviral uses and other effects." *J. Ethnopharmacol.* 1995; 45: 1–18.

Venkateswaran, P., et al. "Effects of an extract from *Phyllanthus niruri* on Hepatitis B and wood chuck hepatitis viruses: *in vitro* and *in vivo* studies." *Proc. Nat. Acad. Sci.* 1987; 84(1): 274–78.

Virusutik, W., et al. "Anti-viral activity of *Phyllanthus niruri* against Hepatitis C." *Malays. Appl. Biol.* 2019: 48(3): 105–111.

Wang, M., et al. "Observations of the efficacy of *Phyllanthus* spp. in treating patients with chronic Hepatitis B." *Zhongguo Zhong Yao Za Zhi.* 1994; 19(12): 750–52.

Wu, W., et al. "Phyllanthin and hypophyllanthin from *Phyllanthus amarus* ameliorates immune-inflammatory response in ovalbumin-induced asthma: role of IgE, Nrf2, iNOs, TNF-α, and IL's." *Immunopharmacol. Immunotoxicol.* 2019 Feb; 41(1): 55–67.

Yuandani, I., et al. "Inhibitory effects of compounds from *Phyllanthus amarus* on nitric oxide production, lymphocyte proliferation, and cytokine release from phagocytes." *Drug Des. Devel. Ther.* 2016 Jun; 10: 1935–45.

Yuandani, I., et al. "Inhibitory effects of standardized extracts of *Phyllanthus amarus* and *Phyllanthus urinaria* and their marker compounds on phagocytic activity of human neutrophils." *Evid. Based Complement. Alternat. Med.* 2013; 2013: 603634.

Chapter 5. The Many Other Benefits of Chanca Piedra

Actions on the Heart (hypotensive, protective)

Amaechina, F., et al. "Hypotensive effect of aqueous extract of the leaves of *Phyllanthus amarus* Schum and Thonn (Euphorbiaceae)." *Acta Pol. Pharm.* 2007 Nov–Dec; 64(6): 547–52.

Amonkan, A., et al. "Comparative effects of two fractions of *Phyllanthus amarus* (Euphorbiaceae) on the blood pressure in rabbit." *Green. J. Med. Sci.* 2013; 3(4): 129–134.

Bello, I., et al. "Blood pressure lowering effect and vascular activity of *Phyllanthus niruri* extract: The role of NO/cGMP signaling pathway and ß-adrenoceptor mediated relaxation of isolated aortic rings." *J. Ethnopharmacol.* 2020 Mar; 250: 112461.

Bharati, D., et al. "Comparative evaluation of antidiabetic antihypertensive activity of *Cynodon dactylon* L. and *Phyllanthus niruri* L in rats with simultaneous type 2 diabetic and hypertension." *Der Pharmacia Lettre.* 2016; 8 (1): 255–263.

Iizuka, T, et al. "Inhibitory effects of methyl brevifolincarboxylate isolated from *Phyllanthus niruri* L. on platelet aggregation." *Biol. Pharm. Bull.* 2007; 30(2): 382–4.

Iizuka, T., et al. "Vasorelaxant effects of methyl brevifolincarboxylate from the leaves of *Phyllanthus niruri.*" *Biol. Pharm. Bull.* 2006; 29(1): 177–9.

Inchoo, M., et al. "Endothelium-independent effects of phyllanthin and hypophyllanthin on vascular tension." *Fitoterapia.* 2011 Dec; 82(8): 1231–6.

Lin, S., et al. "Antioxidant, anti-semicarbazide-sensitive amine oxidase, and anti-hypertensive activities of geraniin isolated from *Phyllanthus urinaria.*" *Food Chem. Toxicol.* 2008; 46(7): 485–92.

Pucci, N., et al. "Effect of *Phyllanthus niruri* on metabolic parameters of patients with kidney stone: a perspective for disease prevention." *Int. Braz. J. Urol.* 2018 Jul–Aug; 44(4): 758–764.

Putakala, M., et al. "Cardioprotective effect of *Phyllanthus amarus* against high fructose diet induced myocardial and aortic stress in rat model." *Biomed. Pharmacother.* 2017 Nov; 95: 1359–1368.

Ramakrishnan, P., et al. "Oral hypoglycaemic effect of *Phyllanthus niruri* leaves." *Indian J. Pharm.* Sci. 1982; 44: 10–12.

Salin, J., et al. "Modulatory effects of stonebreaker (*Phyllanthus amarus*) and bitter gourd (*Momordica charantia*) on enzymes linked with cardiac function in heart tissue of doxorubicin-stressed rats." *Drug. Chem. Toxicol.* 2019 Dec 11: 1–9.

Srividya, N., et al. "Diuretic, hypotensive and hypoglycaemic effect of *Phyllanthus amarus.*" *Indian J. Exp. Biol.* 1995; 33(11): 861–64.

Thippeswamy, A., et al. "Protective role of *Phyllantus niruri* extract in doxorubicin- induced myocardial toxicity in rats." *Indian J. Pharmacol.* 2011 Feb; 43(1): 31–35.

Ueno, H., et al. "Chemical and pharmaceutical studies on medicinal plants in Paraguay, geraniin, an angiotensin-converting enzyme inhibitor from "parapa-rai mi" *Phyllanthus niruri.*" *J. Nat. Prod.* 1988; 51(2): 357–359.

Actions on the Liver (Protective, Detoxifying, Tonic)

Adeneye, A., et al. "Protective effect of the aqueous leaf and seed extract of *Phyllanthus amarus* on gentamicin and acetaminophen-induced nephrotoxic rats." *J. Ethnopharmacol.* 2008 Jul; 118(2): 318–23.

Ali, M., et al. "Selected hepatoprotective herbal medicines: Evidence from ethnomedicinal applications, animal models, and possible mechanism of actions." *Phytother. Res.* 2018 Feb; 32(2): 199–215.

Amin, Z., et al. "Gene expression profiling reveals underlying molecular mechanism of hepatoprotective effect of *Phyllanthus niruri* on thioacetamide-induced hepatotoxicity in Sprague Dawley rats." *BMC Complement. Altern. Med.* 2013 Jul; 13: 160.

Amin, Z., et al. "Protective role of *Phyllanthus niruri* extract against thioacetamide-induced liver cirrhosis in rat model." *Evid. Based Complement. Alternat. Med.* 2012; 2012: 241583.

Appiah-Opong, R., et al. "Interactions between cytochromes P450, glutathione S-transferases and Ghanaian medicinal plants." *Food Chem. Toxicol.* 2008; 46(12): 3598–603.

Bawankule, D., et al. "Protective mechanism of lignans from *Phyllanthus amarus* against galactosamine/ lipopolysaccharide-induced hepatitis: an *in-vivo* and in-silico studies." *Curr. Top. Med. Chem.* 2014; 14(8): 1045–55.

Bedi, O., et al. "Herbal induced hepatoprotection and hepatotoxicity: A critical review." *Indian J. Physiol. Pharmacol.* 2016 Jan–Mar; 60(1): 6–21.

Bhattacharjee, R., et al. "Protein isolate from the herb *Phyllanthus niruri* modulates carbon tetrachloride-induced cytotoxicity in hepatocytes." *Toxicol. Mech. Methods.* 2007; 17(1): 41–7.

Bhattacharjee, R., et al. "The protein fraction of *Phyllanthus niruri* plays a protective role against acetaminophen induced hepatic disorder via its antioxidant properties." *Phytother. Res.* 2006; 20(7): 595–601.

References

Bhattacharjee, R., et al. Protein isolate from the herb, *Phyllanthus niruri* L. (Euphorbiaceae), plays hepatoprotective role against carbon tetrachloride induced liver damage via its antioxidant properties." *Food Chem. Toxicol.* 2007; 45(5): 817–26.

Bhattacharya, S., et al, "A 35 kD *Phyllanthus niruri* protein modulates iron mediated oxidative impairment to hepatocytes via the inhibition of ERKs, p38 MAPKs and activation of PI3k/Akt pathway." *Food Chem. Toxicol.* 2013 Jun; 56: 119–30.

Bhattacharyya, S., et al. "*Phyllanthus niruri* protein suppresses indomethacin mediated hepatic impairments: Its role in Hsp70, HO-1, JNKs and Ca(2+) dependent inflammatory pathways." *Food Chem. Toxicol.* 2017 Apr; 102: 76–92.

Chatterjee, M., et al. "Hepatoprotective effect of aqueous extract of *Phyllanthus niruri* on nimesulide-induced oxidative stress *in vivo*." *Indian J. Biochem. Biophys.* 2006 Oct; 43(5): 299–305.

Chatterjee, M., et al. "Herbal (*Phyllanthus niruri*) protein isolate protects liver from nimesulide induced oxidative stress." *Pathophysiology.* 2006 May; 13(2): 95–102.

Chirdchupunseree, H., et al. "Protective activity of phyllanthin in ethanol-treated primary culture of rat hepatocytes." *J. Ethnopharmacol.* 2010 Mar; 128(1): 172–6.

Dhir, H., et al. "Protection afforded by aqueous extracts of *Phyllanthus* species against cytotoxicity induced by lead and aluminium salts." *Phytother. Res.* 1990; 4(5): 172–76.

Dixit, S., et al. "*Phyllanthus niruri* (Bhumyamalaki) and jaundice in children." *J. Natl. Integ. Med. Ass.* 1982; 25: 269–272.

Ezzat, M., et al. "In-depth hepatoprotective mechanistic study of *Phyllanthus niruri*: *in vitro* and *in vivo* studies and its chemical characterization." *PLoS One.* 2020 Jan; 15(1): e0226185.

Faremi, T., et al. "Hepatoprotective potentials of *Phyllanthus amarus* against ethanol-induced oxidative stress in rats." *Food Chem. Toxicol.* 2008; 46(8): 2658–64.

George, A., et al. "Effects of *Phyllanthus amarus* Phyllpro™ leaves on hangover symptoms: a randomized, double-blind, placebo-controlled crossover study." *Pharm. Biol.* 2019 Dec; 57(1): 145–153.

Guhu, G., et al. "Aqueous extract of *Phyllanthus amarus* inhibits chromium(VI)-induced toxicity in MDA-MB-435S cells." *Food Chem. Toxicol.* 2010 Jan; 48(1): 396–401.

Harikumar, K., et al. "Inhibition of viral carcinogenesis by *Phyllanthus amarus*." *Integrat. Cancer Thera.* 2009; 8(3): 254–260.

Hassan, M., et al. "Efficacy and safety of *Phyllanthus niruri* in non-alcoholic steatohepatitis treatment: pilot study from Malaysia." *J. Pharm. Pract. Commun. Med.* 2017; 3: 131–137.

Hau, D., et al. "*Phyllanthus urinaria* extract attenuates acetaminophen induced hepatotoxicity: involvement of cytochrome P450 CYP2E1." *Phytomedicine.* 2009 Aug; 16(8): 751–60.

Jaleel, C., et al. "NaCl as a physiological modulator of proline metabolism and antioxidant potential in *Phyllanthus amarus.*" *C. R. Biol.* 2007; 330(11): 806–13.

Jeena, K., et al. "Effect of *Emblica officinalis, Phyllanthus amarus* and *Picrorrhiza kurroa* on n-nitrosodiethylamine induced hepatocarcinogenesis." *Cancer Lett.* 1999; 136(1): 11–16.

Jia, R., et al. "Protective action of the phyllanthin against carbon tetrachloride-induced hepatocyte damage in *Cyprinus carpio.*" *In Vitro Cell. Dev. Biol. Anim.* 2016 Jan; 52(1): 1–9.

Khandia, R., et al. "Evaluation of the ameliorative effects of *Phyllanthus niruri* on the deleterious insecticide imidacloprid in the vital organs of chicken embryos." *J. Ayurveda Integr. Med.* 2019 Nov 19. (ahead of print)

Khatoon, S., et al. "Comparative pharmacognostic studies of three *Phyllanthus* species." *J. Ethnopharmacol.* 2006 Mar; 104(1-2): 79–86.

Krithika, R., et al. "Ameliorative potential of *Phyllanthus amarus* against carbon tetrachloride-induced hepatotoxicity." *Acta Pol. Pharm.* 2009 Sep–Oct; 66(5): 579–83.

Krithika, R., et al. "Isolation, characterization and antioxidative effect of phyllanthin against CCl4-induced toxicity in HepG2 cell line." *Chem. Biol. Interact.* 2009 Oct 30; 181(3): 351–8.

Krithika, R., et al. "Mechanism of protective effect of phyllanthin against carbon tetrachloride-induced hepatotoxicity and experimental liver fibrosis in mice." *Toxicol. Mech. Methods.* 2015; 25(9): 708–717.

Krithika, R., et al. "Mitigation of carbon tetrachloride-induced damage by *Phyllanthus amarus* in liver of mice." *Acta Pol. Pharm.* 2009 Jul–Aug; 66(4): 439–44.

Krithika, R., et al. "Phyllanthin inhibits CCl4-mediated oxidative stress and hepatic fibrosis by down-regulating TNF-α/NF-κB, and pro-fibrotic factor TGF-β1 mediating inflammatory signaling." *Toxicol. Ind. Health.* 2016 May; 32(5): 953–60.

Krithika, R., et al. "Phyllanthin of standardized *Phyllanthus amarus* extract attenuates liver oxidative stress in mice and exerts cytoprotective activity on human hepatoma cell line." *J. Clin. Exp. Hepatol.* 2011 Sep; 1(2): 57–67.

Lee, C., et al. "Hepatoprotective effect of *Phyllanthus* in Taiwan on acute liver damage induced by carbon tetrachloride." *Am. J. Chin. Med.* 2006; 34(3): 471–82.

References

Levy, C., et al. "Use of herbal supplements for chronic liver disease." *Clin. Gastroenterol Hepatol.* 2004; 2(11): 947–56.

Londhe, J., et al. "Antioxidant activity of some polyphenol constituents of the medicinal plant *Phyllanthus amarus* Linn." *Redox. Rep.* 2008; 13(5): 199–207.

Londhe, J., et al. "Geraniin and amariin, ellagitannins from *Phyllanthus amarus*, protect liver cells against ethanol induced cytotoxicity." *Fitoterapia.* 2012 Dec; 83(8): 1562–8.

Maity, S., et al. "Bilirubin clearance and antioxidant activities of ethanol extract of *Phyllanthus amarus* root in phenylhydrazine-induced neonatal jaundice in mice." *J. Physiol. Biochem.* 2013 Sep; 69(3): 467–76.

Manjrekar, A., et al. "Effect of *Phyllanthus niruri* Linn. treatment on liver, kidney and testes in CCl4 induced hepatotoxic rats." *Indian J. Exp. Biol.* 2008 Jul; 46(7): 514–20.

Naaz, F., et al. "Hepatoprotective effect of ethanolic extract of *Phyllanthus amarus* Schum. et Thonn. on aflatoxin B1-induced liver damage in mice." *J. Ethnopharmacol.* 2007 Sep; 113(3): 503–9.

Narayanan, B., et al. "Protective effects of *Phyllanthus amarus* on fibrotic markers during alcohol and polyunsaturated fatty acid-induced toxicity." *Toxicol. Mech. Methods.* 2011 Jan; 21(1): 48–52.

Negi, A., et al. "Recent advances in plant hepatoprotectives: a chemical and biological profile of some important leads." *Med. Res. Rev.* 2008 Sep; 28(5): 746–72.

Nipanikar, S., et al. "Pharmacological evaluation of hepatoprotective activity of AHPL/AYTAB/0613 tablet in carbon tetrachloride-, ethanol-, and paracetamol-induced hepatotoxicity models in Wistar albino rats." *Pharmacognosy Res.* 2017 Dec; 9(Suppl 1): S41–S47.

Ooi, K., et al. "Cytotoxic, caspase-3 induction and *in vivo* hepatoprotective effects of phyllanthin, a major constituent of *Phyllanthus niruri*." *J. Funct. Foods.* 2015; 14: 236–243.

Padma, P., et al. "Protective effect of *Phyllanthus fraternus* against carbon tetrachloride-induced mitochondrial dysfunction." *Life Sci.* 1999; 64(25): 2411–17.

Prakash, A., et al. "Comparative hepatoprotective activity of three *Phyllanthus* species, *P. urinaria*, *P. niruri* and *P. simplex*, on carbon tetrachloride induced liver injury in the rat." *Phytother. Res.* 1995; 9(8): 594–96.

Pramyothin, P., et al. "Hepatoprotective activity of *Phyllanthus amarus* Schum. et. Thonn. extract in ethanol treated rats: *in vitro* and *in vivo* studies." *J. Ethnopharmacol.* 2007 Nov; 114(2): 169–73.

Raghdaa, A., et al. "Adipocytokine regulation and antiangiogenic activity underlie the molecular mechanisms of therapeutic effects of *Phyllanthus niruri* against non-alcoholic fatty liver disease." *Nutrients.* 2018 Aug 9; 10(8).

Raghdaa, A., et al. "*Phyllanthus niruri* standardized extract alleviates the progression of non-alcoholic fatty liver disease and decreases atherosclerotic risk in Sprague-Dawley rats." *Nutrients*. 2017 Jul 18; 9(7).

Rai, V., et al. "Chromium-induced changes in ultramorphology and secondary metabolites of *Phyllanthus amarus* Schum & Thonn. – an hepatoprotective plant." *Environ. Monit. Assess.* 2008 Dec; 147(1-3): 307–15.

Rajeshkumar, N., et al. "*Phyllanthus amarus* extract administration increases the life span of rats with hepatocellular carcinoma." *J. Ethnopharmacol.* 2000 Nov; 73(1-2): 215–19.

Reddy, B., et al. "A natural small molecule inhibitor corilagin blocks HCV replication and modulates oxidative stress to reduce liver damage." *Antiviral Res.* 2018 Feb; 150: 47–59.

Sabir, S., et al. "Water-extractable phytochemicals from *Phyllanthus niruri* exhibit distinct *in vitro* antioxidant and *in vivo* hepatoprotective activity against paracetamol-induced liver damage in mice." *Food Chem.* 2008; 111: 845–851.

Saravanan, M., et al. "*In-vitro* qualitative and quantitative analysis of certain nutraceuticals as diuretic and antioxidant for hepatobiliary disorders (HBD)." *Int. J. Pharma Sci. Res.* 2014 Dec; 5(2): 896–902.

Sarkar, M., et al. "Hepatocytes are protected by herb *Phyllanthus niruri* protein isolate against thioacetamide toxicity." *Pathophysiology*. 2007 Oct; 14(2): 113–20.

Sethiya, N., et al, "Antioxidant and hepatoprotective effects of mixed micellar lipid formulation of phyllanthin and piperine in carbon tetrachloride-induced liver injury in rodents." *Food Funct.* 2015 Nov; 6(11): 3593–3603.

Shanmugam, B., et al. "Exploratory studies of (-)-epicatechin, a bioactive compound of *Phyllanthus niruri*, on the antioxidant enzymes and oxidative stress markers in D-galactosamine-induced hepatitis in rats: A study with reference to clinical prospective." *Pharmacogn. Mag.* 2017 Jan; 13(Suppl 1): S56–S62.

Sharma, S., et al. "Hepatoprotective activity of the *Phyllanthus* species on tert-butyl hydroperoxide (t-BH)-induced cytotoxicity in HepG2 cells." *Pharmacogn. Mag.* 2011 Jul; 7(27): 229–33.

Shen, B., et al. "*Phyllanthus urinaria* ameliorates the severity of nutritional steatohepatitis both *in vitro* and *in vivo*." *Hepatology*. 2008 Feb; 47(2): 473–83.

Singh, M., et al. "Preclinical hepatoprotective effect of herbalism against ethanol induced hepatotoxicity: A review." *Curr. Drug. Metab.* 2018; 19(12): 1002–1011.

Sreenivasa, R. "Experimental production of liver damage and its protection with *Phyllanthus niruri* and *Capparis spinosa* (both ingredients of LIV52) in white albino rats." *Probe* 1985; 24(2): 117–19.

Srirama, R., et al. "Hepatoprotective activity of Indian *Phyllanthus*." *Pharm. Biol.* 2012 Aug; 50(8): 948–53.

Stickel, F., et al. "Herbal medicine in the treatment of liver diseases." *Dig. Liver Dis.* 2007; 39(4): 293–304.

Suganya, S., et al. "Molecular docking studies of potential inhibition of the alcohol dehydrogenase enzyme by phyllanthin, hypophyllanthin and gallic acid." *Crit. Rev. Eukaryot. Gene Expr.* 2019; 29(4): 287–294.

Syamasundar, K., et al. "Antihepatotoxic principles of *Phyllanthus niruri* herbs." *J. Ethnopharmacol.* 1985; 14(1): 41–4.

Thabrew, M., et al. "Phytogenic agents in the therapy of liver disease." *Phytother. Res.* 1996; 10(6): 461–67.

Thakur, J., et al. "Enhancing hepatoprotective bioactives of *Phyllanthus amarus* through immobilization by growth promoters and media changes." *Indian J. Pharm. Sci.* 2011 May; 73(3): 271–5.

Umarani, D., et al. "Ethanol induced metabolic alterations and the effect of *Phyllanthus niruri* in their reversal." *Ancient Sci. Life* 1985; 4(3): 174–80.

Wong, V., et al. "Treatment of nonalcoholic steatohepatitis with *Phyllanthus urinaria* - A randomized trial." *J. Gastroenterol. Hepatol.* 2013 Jan; 28(1): 57–62.

Xu, M., et al. "Phenolic antioxidants from the whole plant of *Phyllanthus urinaria.*" *Chem. Biodivers.* 2007 Sep; 4(9): 2246–52.

Yadav, N., et al. "Synergistic effect of silymarin and standardized extract of *Phyllanthus amarus* against CCl4-induced hepatotoxicity in *Rattus norvegicus.*" *Phytomedicine.* 2008 Dec; 15(12): 1053–61.

Zhang, R., et al. "Corilagin alleviates nonalcoholic fatty liver disease in high-fat diet-induced C57BL/6 mice by ameliorating oxidative stress and restoring autophagic flux." *Front. Pharmacol.* 2020 Feb; 10: 1693.

Anti-Aging and AGE-Inhibitor Actions

Adedapo, A., et al. "The evaluation of the hypoglycemic effect of soft drink leaf extract of *Phyllanthus amarus* (Euphorbiaceae) in rats." *J. Basic Clin. Physiol. Pharmacol.* 2014 Feb; 25(1): 47–57.

Adeneye, A. "The leaf and seed aqueous extract of *Phyllanthus amarus* improves insulin resistance diabetes in experimental animal studies." *J. Ethnopharmacol.* 2012 Dec 18; 144(3): 705–11.

Adeneye, A., et al. "Hypoglycemic and hypocholesterolemic activities of the aqueous leaf and seed extract of *Phyllanthus amarus* in mice." *Fitoterapia.* 2006 Dec; 77(7-8): 511–4.

Ali, H., et al. "Alpha-amylase inhibitory activity of some Malaysian plants used to treat diabetes; with particular reference to *Phyllanthus amarus.*" *J. Ethnopharmacol.* 2006 Oct; 107(3): 449–55.

Garay, M., et al. "Extracts of *Phyllanthus niruri*." U.S. Patent # 8916209B2. Dec 2014 Assigned to Johnson & Johnson Consumer Companies, Inc.

Okoli, C., et al. "Studies on the possible mechanisms of antidiabetic activity of extract of aerial parts of *Phyllanthus niruri*." *Pharm. Biol.* 2011 Mar; 49(3): 248–55.

Rao, A., et al. "Aldose reductase inhibitory and antiglycation activities of four medicinal plant standardized extracts and their main constituents for the prevention of diabetic complications." *Ethiop. Pharm. J.* 2015; 31: 1–14.

Sompong, W., et al. "Inhibitory effect of herbal medicines and their trapping abilities against methylglyoxal-derived advanced glycation end-products." *BMC Complement. Altern. Med.* 2015 Oct; 15: 394.

Anti-Diabetic and Anti-Cholesterol Actions

Beidokhti, M., et al. "Investigation of antidiabetic potential of *Phyllanthus niruri* L. using assays for α-glucosidase, muscle glucose transport, liver glucose production, and adipogenesis." *Biochem. Biophys. Res. Commun.* 2017 Nov; 493(1): 869–874.

Feliciana, A., et al. "Effect of *Phyllanthus niruri* extract on low density lipoprotein of dyslipidemic white rats (*Rattus norvegicus*)." *J. Herbal Med.* 2019; 5(2): 6.

Giribabu, N., et al. "Aqueous extract of *Phyllanthus niruri* leaves displays *in vitro* antioxidant activity and prevents the elevation of oxidative stress in the kidney of streptozotocin-induced diabetic male rats." *Evid. Based Complement. Alternat. Med.* 2014; 2014: 834815.

Giribabu, N., et al. "*Phyllanthus niruri* leaves aqueous extract improves kidney functions, ameliorates kidney oxidative stress, inflammation, fibrosis and apoptosis and enhances kidney cell proliferation in adult male rats with Diabetes mellitus." *J. Ethnopharmacol.* 2017 Jun; 205: 123–137.

Gunawan-Puteri, M., et al. "Alpha-amylase inhibitors from an Indonesian medicinal herb, *Phyllanthus urinaria*." *J. Sci. Food Agric.* 2012 Feb; 92(3): 606–9.

Jagtap, S., et al. "Protective effects of phyllanthin, a lignan from *Phyllanthus amarus*, against progression of high fat diet induced metabolic disturbances in mice." *RSC Adv.* 2016; 6: 58343–58353.

Karuna, R., et al. "Protective effects of *Phyllanthus amarus* aqueous extract against renal oxidative stress in streptozotocin-induced diabetic rats." *Indian J. Pharmacol.* 2011 Jul; 43(4): 414–8.

Khanna, A., et al. "Lipid lowering activity of *Phyllanthus niruri* in hyperlipemic rats." *J. Ethnopharmacol.* 2002; 82(1): 19–22.

Kumar, A., et al. "Effect of methanolic extract of *Phyllanthus niruri* on leptin level in animal model of Diabetes mellitus." *Biomed. Pharmacol. J.* 2019 Mar; 12(1): 57–63.

Latha, P., et al. "Protective effect of *Phyllanthus niruri* on alcohol and heated sunflower oil induced hyperlipidemia in Wistar rats." *Toxicol. Mech. Methods.* 2010 Oct; 20(8): 498–503.

Luliana, S., et al. "Total flavonoid contents and in silico study of flavonoid compounds from Meniran (*Phyllanthus niruri* L.) towards alpha-amylase and alpha-glucosidase enzymes." *Pharmaciana.* 2019 May; 9(1): 1–10.

Mediani, A., "Metabolic and biochemical changes in streptozotocin induced obese-diabetic rats treated with *Phyllanthus niruri* extract." *J. Pharm. Biomed. Anal.* 2016 Sep; 128: 302–312.

Modak, M., et al. "Indian herbs and herbal drugs used for the treatment of diabetes." *J. Clin. Biochem. Nutr.* 2007 May; 40(3): 163–73.

Nandini, H., et al. "Action of corilagin on hyperglycemia, hyperlipidemia and oxidative stress in streptozotocin-induced diabetic rats." *Chem. Biol. Interact.* 2019 Feb; 299: 186–193.

Okoli, C., et al. "Studies on the possible mechanisms of antidiabetic activity of extract of aerial parts of *Phyllanthus niruri.*" *Pharm. Biol.* 2011 Mar; 49(3): 248–55.

Patel, K., et al. "Effect of Atibalamula and Bhumyamalaki on thirty-three patients of diabetic neuropathy." *Ayu.* 2011 Jul; 32(3): 353–6.

Putakala, M., et al. "Beneficial effects of *Phyllanthus amarus* against high fructose diet induced insulin resistance and hepatic oxidative stress in male Wistar Rats." *Appl. Biochem. Biotechnol.* 2017 Nov; 183(3): 744–764.

Ramakrishnan, P., et al. "Oral hypoglycaemic effect of *Phyllanthus niruri* (Linn.) leaves." *Indian J. Pharm. Sci.* 1982; 44(1): 10–12.

Raphael, K., et al. "Hypoglycemic effect of methanol extract of *Phyllanthus amarus* Schum & Thonn on alloxan induced diabetes mellitus in rats and its relation with antioxidant potential." *Indian J. Exp. Biol.* 2002; 40(8): 905–9.

Shimizu, M., et al. "Studies on aldose reductase inhibitors from natural products. II. Active components of a Paraguayan crude drug, 'paraparai mi,' *Phyllanthus niruri.*" *Chem. Pharm. Bull.* (Tokyo) 1989; 37(9): 2531–32.

Sompong, W., et al. "The inhibitory activity of herbal medicines on the keys enzymes and steps related to carbohydrate and lipid digestion." *BMC Complement. Altern. Med.* 2016 Nov; 16(1): 439.

Srividya, N., et al. "Diuretic, hypotensive and hypoglycaemic effect of *Phyllanthus amarus.*" *Indian J. Exp. Biol.* 1995; 33(11): 861–64.

Sutrisna, E., et al. "Antidiabetic potencies of *Phyllanthus niruri* Linn and thin-layer chromatography profile." *Drug Invention Today.* 2019 Oct; 11(10): 2339–2341.

Tamil, I., et al. "*In vitro* study on alpha-amylase inhibitory activity of an Indian medicinal plant, *Phyllanthus amarus.*" *Indian J. Pharmacol.* 2010 Oct; 42(5): 280–2.

Trinh, B., et al. "Screening for potential α-glucosidase and α-amylase inhibitory constituents from selected Vietnamese plants used to treat type 2 diabetes." *J. Ethnopharmacol.* 2016 Jun; 186: 189–195.

Umarani, D., et al. "Ethanol induced metabolic alterations and the effect of *Phyllanthus niruri* in their reversal." *Ancient Sci. Life* 1985; 4(3): 174–80.

Umbare, R., et al. "Quality evaluation of *Phyllanthus amarus* (Schumach) leaves extract for its hypolipidemic activity." *Biol. Med.* 2009; 1(4): 28–33.

Zar, C., et al. "Potential effect of herbs on diabetic hypertension: alternative medicine treatment modalities." *Clin. Ter.* 2013; 164(6): 529–35.

Zin, M., et al. "Anti-diabetic potential of peptide from *P. niruri* reveals through carbohydrate hydrolyzing enzyme inhibition assay." *Sci. Herit. J.* 2019; 3(1): 17–19.

Anti-Inflammatory and Pain-Relieving Actions

Adedapo, A., et al. "Anti-inflammatory and antinociceptive activities of the aqueous leaf extract of *Phyllanthus amarus* Schum (Euphorbiaceae) in some laboratory animals." *J. Basic Clin. Physiol. Pharmacol.* 2015 Jan; 26(1): 89–94.

Alagan, A., et al. "Protective effects of *Phyllanthus amarus* against lipopolysaccharide- induced neuroinflammation and cognitive impairment in rats." *Front Pharmacol.* 2019 Jun; 10: 632.

Alam, J., et al. "Suppressive effects of the standardized extract of *Phyllanthus amarus* on type II collagen-induced rheumatoid arthritis in Sprague Dawley rats." *Curr. Phar. Biotechnol.* 2018; 19(14): 1156–1169.

Bhat, S., et al. "Preclinical screening of *Phyllanthus amarus* ethanolic extract for its analgesic and antimicrobial activity." *Pharmacognosy Res.* 2014 Oct–Dec; 7(4): 378–84.

Buddhachat, K., et al. "*In vitro* chondroprotective potential of extracts obtained from various *Phyllanthus* species." *Planta Med.* 2017 Jan; 83(1-02): 87–96.

Chopade, A., et al. "Molecular docking studies of phytocompounds from the *Phyllanthus* species as potential chronic pain modulators." *Sci. Pharm.* 2014 Nov; 83(2): 243–67.

Chopade, A., et al. "Pain modulation by lignans (phyllanthin and hypophyllanthin) and tannin (corilagin) rich extracts of *Phyllanthus amarus* in carrageenan-induced thermal and mechanical chronic muscle hyperalgesia." *Phytother. Res.* 2015 Aug; 29(8): 1202–10.

Dirjomuljono, M., et al. "Symptomatic treatment of acute tonsillo-pharyngitis patients with a combination of *Nigella sativa* and *Phyllanthus niruri* extract." *Int. J. Clin. Pharmacol. Ther.* 2008; 46(6): 295–306.

Fang, S., et al. "Anti-oxidant and inflammatory mediator's growth inhibitory effects of compounds isolated from *Phyllanthus urinaria*." *J. Ethnopharmacol.* 2008 Mar; 116(2): 333–40.

References

Forouzanfar, F., et al. "Medicinal herbs in the treatment of neuropathic pain: a review." *Iran J. Basic Med. Sci.* 2018 Apr; 21(4): 347–358.

Gebhardt, R., et al. "Use of *Phyllanthus* for treating chronic inflammatory and fibrotic processes." U.S. Patent # 6586015B1. July 2003. Assigned to Phytrix AG.

Harikrishnan, H., "Phyllanthin from *Phyllanthus amarus* inhibits LPS-induced proinflammatory responses in U937 macrophages via downregulation of NF-κB/MAPK/PI3K-Akt signaling pathways." *Phytother. Res.* 2018 Dec; 32(12): 2510–2519.

Harikrishnan, H., et al. "Anti-inflammatory effects of *Phyllanthus amarus* Schum. & Thonn. through inhibition of NF-κB, MAPK, and PI3K-Akt signaling pathways in LPS-induced human macrophages." *BMC Complement. Altern. Med.* 2018 Jul 25; 18(1): 224.

Iranloye, B., et al. "Analgesic activity of aqueous leaf extract of *Phyllanthus amarus.*" *Afr. J. Med. Med. Sci.* 2011 Mar; 40(1): 47–50.

Kassuya, C., et al. "Antiinflammatory and antiallodynic actions of the lignan niranthin isolated from *Phyllanthus amarus*. Evidence for interaction with platelet activating factor receptor." *Eur. J. Pharmacol.* 2006 Sep; 546(1–3): 182–8.

Kassuya, C., et al. "Anti-inflammatory properties of extracts, fractions and lignans isolated from *Phyllanthus amarus.*" *Planta Med.* 2005; 71(8): 721–6.

Kiemer, A., et al. "*Phyllanthus amarus* has anti-inflammatory potential by inhibition of iNOS, COX-2, and cytokines via the NF-kappaB pathway." *J. Hepatol.* 2003; 38(3): 289–97.

Lai, C., et al. "Inhibition of *Helicobacter pylori*-induced inflammation in human gastric epithelial AGS cells by *Phyllanthus urinaria* extracts." *J. Ethnopharmacol.* 2008 Aug; 118(3): 522–6.

Miguel, O., et al. "Chemical and preliminary analgesic evaluation of geraniin and furosin isolated from *Phyllanthus sellowianus.*" *Planta Med.* 1996; 62(2): 146–49.

Moreira, J., et al. "Anti-hyperalgesic activity of corilagin, a tannin isolated from *Phyllanthus niruri* L. (Euphorbiaceae)." *J. Ethnopharmacol.* 2013 Mar; 146(1): 318–23.

Mostofa, R., et al. "Evaluation of anti-inflammatory and gastric anti-ulcer activity of *Phyllanthus niruri* L. (Euphorbiaceae) leaves in experimental rats." *BMC Complement. Altern. Med.* 2017 May 16; 17(1): 267.

Obidike, I., et al. "The anti-inflammatory and antinociceptive properties of the chloroform fraction from *Phyllanthus niruri* plant is mediated via the peripheral nervous system." *J. Diet. Suppl.* 2010 Dec; 7(4): 341–50.

Ofuegbe, S., et al. "Anti-inflammatory and analgesic activities of the methanol leaf extract of *Phyllanthus amarus* in some laboratory animals." *J. Basic Clin. Physiol. Pharmacol.* 2014 May; 25(2): 175–80.

Okoli, C., et al. "Extracts of *Phyllanthus niruri* aerial parts suppress acute and chronic inflammation in murine models." *J. Herbs Spices Med. Plants.* 2014; 20(3): 256–268.

Pradit. W., et al. "Chondroprotective potential of *Phyllanthus amarus* Schum. & Thonn. in experimentally induced cartilage degradation in the explants culture model." *In Vitro Cell. Dev. Biol. Anim.* 2015 Apr; 51(4): 336–44.

Roengrit, T., et al. "Antioxidant and anti-nociceptive effects of *Phyllanthus amarus* on improving exercise recovery in sedentary men: a randomized crossover (double-blind) design." *J. Int. Soc. Sports Nutr.* 2014 Mar; 11(1): 9.

Santos, A., et al. "Analgesic effects of callus culture extracts from selected species of *Phyllanthus* in mice." *J. Pharm. Pharmacol.* 1994; 46(9): 755–59.

Santos, A., et al. "Analysis of the mechanisms underlying the antinociceptive effect of the extracts of plants from the genus *Phyllanthus*." *Gen. Pharmacol.* 1995; 26(7): 1499–1506.

Santos, A., et al. "Antinociceptive properties of extracts of new species of plants of the genus *Phyllanthus* (Euphorbiaceae)." *J. Ethnopharmacol.* 2000; 72(1/2): 229–38.

Santos, A., et al. "Further studies on the antinociceptive action of the hydroalcohlic extracts from plants of the genus *Phyllanthus*." *J. Pharm. Pharmacol.* 1995; 47(1): 66–71.

Sutrisna, E., et al. "Anti-inflammatory effect of *Phyllanthus niruri* L. from Indonesia; Preclinical Study." *Pharmacog. J.* 2019 Nov; 11(6): 1347–50.

Wu, W., et al. "Phyllanthin and hypophyllanthin from *Phyllanthus amarus* ameliorates immune-inflammatory response in ovalbumin-induced asthma: role of IgE, Nrf2, iNOs, TNF-α, and IL's." *Immunopharmacol. Immunotoxicol.* 2019 Feb; 41(1): 55–67.

Anti-Osteoporosis Actions

Li, K., et al. "Geraniin promotes osteoblast proliferation and differentiation via the activation of Wnt/β-catenin pathway." *Biomed. Pharmacother.* 2018 Mar; 99: 319–324.

Mo, J., et al. "Geraniin promotes osteogenic differentiation of bone marrow mesenchymal stem cells (BMSCs) via activating ß-catenin: a comparative study between BMSCs from normal and osteoporotic rats." *J. Nat. Med.* 2019; 73: 262–272.

Antioxidant Actions

Ahmeda, A., et al. "Antioxidant properties of *Phyllanthus niruri* (Dukung anak) extracts." *Asian. J. Food Ag-Ind.* 2009; 2(3): 373–381.

Akporowhe, S., et al. "*Phyllanthus amarus* augments the serum antioxidant capacity and invigorates the blood in experimental mice." *Biosci. Biotechnol. Res. Commun.* 2016; 9: 15–18.

Balaguru, S., "Assessment of nutritional composition and antioxidant activity of edible herbs *Solanum nigrum* and *Phyllanthus niruri*." *Int. J. Res. Ins.* 2019 Apr; 6(1): 1–12.

Bhattacharjee, R., et al. "The protein fraction of *Phyllanthus niruri* plays a protective role against acetaminophen induced hepatic disorder via its antioxidant properties." *Phytother. Res.* 2006 May; 20: 595–601.

Colpo, E., et al. "Antioxidant effects of *Phyllanthus niruri* tea on healthy subjects." *Asian Pac. J. Trop. Med.* 2014 Feb; 7(2): 113–8.

Da'i, M., et al. "Antioxidant activity of *Phyllanthus niruri* L. herbs: *in vitro* and *in vivo* models and isolation of active compound." *Natl. J. Physiol. Pharm. Pharmacol.* 2016; 6(1): 32–37.

Devi, S., et al. "*In-vitro* antioxidant activities of methanolic extract of whole plant of *Phyllanthus amarus* (Euphorbiaceae)." *Int. J. Bot. Study.* 2016 Mar; 1(3): 30–32.

Devi, S., et al. "*In vitro* antioxidant potential of methanolic extract of whole plant of *Phyllanthus amarus* Schum (Euphorbiaceae)." *Int. J. Bot. Stud.* 2017; 2: 100–102.

Kaur, R., et al. "Phytochemical screening of *Phyllanthus niruri* collected from Kerala region and its antioxidant and antimicrobial potentials." *J. Pharm. Sci. & Res.* 2017; 9(8): 1312–1316.

Londhe, J., et al. "Antioxidant activity of some polyphenol constituents of the medicinal plant *Phyllanthus amarus* Linn." *Redox Report.* 2008; 13(5): 199–207.

Mahdi, E., et al. "Identification of phenolic compounds and assessment of *in vitro* antioxidants activity of 30% ethanolic extracts derived from two *Phyllanthus* species indigenous to Malaysia." *Afr. J. Pharm. Pharmacol.* 2011 Nov; 5(17): 1967–1978.

Maity, S., et al. "Evaluation of antioxidant activity and characterization of phenolic constituents of *Phyllanthus amarus* root." *J. Agric. Food Chem.* 2013 Apr; 61(14): 3443–50.

Mehta, M., et al. "Phytochemical and antioxidants profiling of *Phyllanthus niruri*: a hepatoprotective plant." *World J. Pharm. Pharmaceut. Sci.* 2019 July; 8(8): 1117–1127.

Menendez-Perdomo, I., et al. "Antioxidant, photoprotective and antimutagenic properties of *Phyllanthus spp.* from Cuban flora." *J. Pharm. Pharmacogn. Res.* 2017; 5: 251–261.

Navarro, M., et al. "Proanthocyanidin characterization, antioxidant and cytotoxic activities of three plants commonly used in traditional medicine in Costa Rica: *Petiveria alliaceae* L., *Phyllanthus niruri* L. and *Senna reticulata* Willd." *Plants.*" 2017 Oct 19; 6(4): 50.

Nguyen, V., et al. "Physicochemical properties, antioxidant and cytotoxic activities of crude extracts and fractions from *Phyllanthus amarus.*" *Medicines.* 2017 Jun 18; 4(2).

Nguyen, V., et al. "Influence of solvents and novel extraction methods on bioactive compounds and antioxidant capacity of *Phyllanthus amarus.*" *Chem. Pap.* 2016; 70: 556–566.

Rajamanickam, G., et al. "Identification and comparative study of *in vitro* antioxidant potential of fractionated hydroalcoholic extract of *Phyllanthus niruri* Linn." *Euro. J. Adv. Chem. Res.* 2020 Jan. 1(1): 1–7.

Roengrit, T., et al, "Antioxidant effect of *Phyllanthus amarus* after moderate-intensity exercise in sedentary males: A randomized crossover (double-blind) study." *J. Phys. Ther. Sci.* 2015 Apr; 27(4): 1181–6.

Roengrit, T., et al. "Antioxidant and anti-nociceptive effects of *Phyllanthus amarus* on improving exercise recovery in sedentary men: a randomized crossover (double-blind) design." *J. Int. Soc. Sports Nutr.* 2014 Mar 17; 11(1): 9.

Rusmana, D., et al. "Antioxidant activity of *Phyllanthus niruri* extract, rutin and quercetin." *Indones. Biomed. J.* 2017 Aug; 9(2): 84–90.

Sabir, S., et al. "Water-extractable phytochemicals from *Phyllanthus niruri* exhibit distinct *in vitro* antioxidant and *in vivo* hepatoprotective activity against paracetamol-induced liver damage in mice." *Food Chem.* 2008; 111: 845–851.

Shanmugam, B., et al. "Exploratory studies of (-)-epicatechin, a bioactive compound of *Phyllanthus niruri,* on the antioxidant enzymes and oxidative stress markers in D-galactosamine-induced hepatitis in rats: A study with reference to clinical prospective." *Pharmacogn. Mag.* 2017 Jan; 13(Suppl 1): S56–S62.

Singh, R., et al. "Antioxidant activity of ethanolic and aqueous extract of *Phyllanthus niruri—In vitro.*" *World J. Pharm. Pharm. Sci.* 2016; 5: 1994–2000.

Than, N., et al. "Niruriflavone, a new antioxidant flavone sulfonic acid from *Phyllanthus niruri.*" *Zeitschrift Naturforschung.* 2006 Jan; 61(1): 57–60.

Zane, S., et al. "Antioxidant activity, total phenolic content and total flavonoid content of water and methanol extracts of *Phyllanthus* species from Malaysia." *Pharmacog. J.* 2018 Jul-Aug; 10(4): 677–68.

Cellular-Protective Antioxidant Actions

Adedayo, B., et al. "Effect of *Andrographis paniculata* and *Phyllanthus amarus* leaf extracts on selected biochemical indices in *Drosophila melanogaster* model of neurotoxicity." *Drug. Chem. Toxicol.* 2020 Jan 3: 1–10.

Ahmad, S., et al. "Cancer ameliorating potential of *Phyllanthus amarus: in vivo* and *in vitro* studies against Aflatoxin B1 toxicity." *Egypt. J. Med. Human Genetics.* 2015; 16(4): 343–353.

References

Alagan, A., et al. "*Phyllanthus amarus* protects against spatial memory impairment induced by lipopolysaccharide in mice." *Bioinformation.* 2019 Aug; 15(8): 535–541.

Alagan, A., et al. "Protective effects of *Phyllanthus amarus* against lipopolysaccharide- induced neuroinflammation and cognitive impairment in rats." *Front. Pharmacol.* 2019 Jun; 10: 632.

Ambali, S., et al. "Alleviating effect of *Phyllanthus niruri* on sensorimotor and cognitive changes induced by subacute chlorpyrifos exposure in Wistar rats." *Am. J. Med. Med. Sci.* 2012; 2(3): 50–58.

Berezi, E., et al. "Gastroprotective potentials of aqueous leaf extracts of *Phyllanthus amarus* on ibuprofen-induced ulcer in Wistar rats." *Int. J. Adv. Res. Biol. Sci.* 2017; 4: 138–146.

Bhattacharyya, S., et al. "Amelioration of aspirin induced oxidative impairment and apoptotic cell death by a novel antioxidant protein molecule isolated from the herb *Phyllanthus niruri*." *PLoS One.* 2014 Feb 19; 9(2): e89026.

Bongu, S., et al. "Protective role of aqueous extract of *Phyllanthus amarus* on oxidative stress in pancreas of streptozotocin induced diabetic male Wistar rats." *J. Exp. Appl. Anim. Sci.* 2016; 2: 23–30.

Boonyong, C., et al. "Natural polyphenols prevent indomethacin-induced and diclofenac-induced Caco-2 cell death by reducing endoplasmic reticulum stress regardless of their direct reactive oxygen species scavenging capacity." *J. Pharm. Pharmacol.* 2020 Jan 10: 13227. (ahead of print)

Chularojmontri, L., et al. "Cytoprotective role of *Phyllanthus urinaria* L. and glutathione-S transferase Pi in doxorubicin-induced toxicity in H9c2 cells." *J. Med. Assoc. Thai.* 2009 Jun; 92 Suppl 3: S43–51.

de Melo, M., et al. "Spray-dried extract of *Phyllanthus niruri* L. reduces mucosal damage in rats with intestinal inflammation." *J. Pharm. Pharmacol.* 2015 Aug; 67(8): 1107–18.

Devi, P. "Radioprotective effect of *Phyllanthus niruri* on mouse chromosomes." *Curr. Sci.* 2000; 78(10): 1245–47.

Giribabu, N., et al. "Aqueous extract of *Phyllanthus niruri* leaves displays *in vitro* antioxidant activity and prevents the elevation of oxidative stress in the kidney of streptozotocin-induced diabetic male rats." *Evid. Based Complement. Alternat. Med.* 2014; 2014: 834815.

Guha, G., et al. "Aqueous extract of *Phyllanthus amarus* inhibits chromium(VI)-induced toxicity in MDA-MB-435S cells." *Food Chem. Toxicol.* 2010 Jan; 48(1): 396–401.

Guha G., et al. "Antimycin A-induced mitochondrial apoptotic cascade is mitigated by phenolic constituents of *Phyllanthus amarus* aqueous extract in Hep3B cells." *Food. Chem. Toxicol.* 2010; 48(12): 3449–3457.

Harikumar, K., et al. "An extract of *Phyllanthus amarus* protects mouse chromosomes and intestine from radiation induced damages." *J. Radiat. Res.* 2007 Nov; 48(6): 469–76.

Jagetia, G. "Radioprotective potential of plants and herbs against the effects of ionizing radiation." *J. Clin. Biochem. Nutr.* 2007 Mar; 40(2): 74–81.

Jin, F., et al. "Anti-inflammatory and anti-oxidative effects of corilagin in a rat model of acute cholestasis." *BMC. Gastroenterol.* 2013; 13: 79.

Karuna, R., et al. "Protective effects of *Phyllanthus amarus* aqueous extract against renal oxidative stress in streptozotocin-induced diabetic rats." *Indian J. Pharmacol.* 2011 Jul; 43(4): 414–8.

Khandia, R., et al. "Evaluation of the ameliorative effects of *Phyllanthus niruri* on the deleterious insecticide imidacloprid in the vital organs of chicken embryos." *J. Ayurveda Integr. Med.* 2019 Nov 19. (ahead of print)

Klein-Junior, L., et al. "The protective potential of *Phyllanthus niruri* and corilagin on gastric lesions induced in rodents by different harmful agents." *Planta Med.* 2017 Jan; 83(1-02): 30–39.

Koay, Y., et al. "Isocorilagin, a cholinesterase inhibitor from *Phyllanthus niruri*." *Nat. Prod. Commun.* 2014 Apr; 9(4): 515-7.

Kumar, K., et al. "Chemoprotective activity of an extract of *Phyllanthus amarus* against cyclophosphamide induced toxicity in mice." *Phytomedicine.* 2005; 12(6-7): 494–500.

Londhe, J., et al. "Radioprotective properties of polyphenols from *Phyllanthus amarus* Linn." *J. Radiat. Res.* 2009 Jul; 50(4): 303–9.

Mostofa, R., et al. "Evaluation of anti-inflammatory and gastric anti-ulcer activity of *Phyllanthus niruri* L. (Euphorbiaceae) leaves in experimental rats." *BMC Complement. Altern. Med.* 2017 May; 17(1): 267.

Putakala, M., et al. "Cardioprotective effect of *Phyllanthus amarus* against high fructose diet induced myocardial and aortic stress in rat model." *Biomed. Pharmacother.* 2017 Nov; 95(): 1359–1368.

Raphael, K., et al. "Inhibition of experimental gastric lesion and inflammation by *Phyllanthus amarus* extract." *J. Ethnopharmacol.* 2003; 87(2-3): 193–7.

Sarkar, M., et al. "Prevention of tertiary butyl hydroperoxide induced oxidative impairment and cell death by a novel antioxidant protein molecule isolated from the herb, *Phyllanthus niruri*." *Toxicol. In Vitro.* 2010 Sep; 24(6): 1711–9.

Sharma, P., et al. "Chemopreventive effect of papillomagenesis in Swiss albino mice." *Int. J. Biol. Med. Res.* 2010; 1(4): 158–16.

Sharma, P., et al. "Protective effect of *Phyllanthus niruri* on DMBA/croton Oil mediated carcinogenic response and oxidative damage in accordance to histopathological studies in skin of mice." *J. Nat. Sci. Res.* 2011; 1(4): 16–28.

Singh, H., et al. "Protective role of *Phyllanthus fraternus* in alloxan-induced diabetes in rats." *J. Ayurveda Integr. Med.* 2020 Feb; (ahead of print)

Souza, C., et al. "Compounds extracted from *Phyllanthus* and *Jatropha elliptica* inhibit the binding of [3H]glutamate and [3H]GMP-PNP in rat cerebral cortex membrane." *Neurochem. Res.* 2000; 25(2): 211–15.

Thakur, I., et al. "Protection against radiation clastogenecity in mouse bone marrow by *Phyllanthus niruri.*" *Indian J. Exp. Biol.* 2011 Sep; 49(9): 704–10.

Thippeswamy, A., et al. "Protective role of *Phyllanthus niruri* extract in doxorubicin-induced myocardial toxicity in rats." *Indian J. Pharmacol.* 2011 Feb; 43(1): 31–5.

Tong, F., et al. "Corilagin attenuates radiation-induced brain injury in mice." *Mol. Neurobiol.* 2016 Dec; 53(10): 6982–6996.

Cytotoxic and Anticancer Actions

Araujo, R., et al. "A dry extract of *Phyllanthus niruri* protects normal cells and induces apoptosis in human liver carcinoma cells." *Exp. Biol. Med.* 2012 Nov; 237(11): 1281–8.

Araujo, R., et al. "Growth inhibitory effects of *Phyllanthus niruri* extracts in combination with cisplatin on cancer cell lines." *World J. Gastroenterol.* 2012 Aug; 18(31): 4162–6168.

Guhu, G., et al. "Antimycin A-induced mitochondrial apoptotic cascade is mitigated by phenolic constituents of *Phyllanthus amarus* aqueous extract in Hep3B cells." *Food Chem. Toxicol.* 2010 Dec; 48(12): 3449–57.

Guo, J., et al. "Effect of *Phyllanthus amarus* extract on 5-fluorouracil-induced perturbations in ribonucleotide and deoxyribonucleotide pools in HepG2 cell line." *Molecules.* 2016 Sep; 21(9): E1254.

Gupta, A., et al. "Corilagin in Cancer: A critical evaluation of anticancer activities and molecular mechanisms." *Molecules.* 2019 Sep; 24(18): E3399.

Harikrishnan, H., et al. "Modulation of cell signaling pathways by *Phyllanthus amarus* and its major constituents: potential role in the prevention and treatment of inflammation and cancer." *Inflammopharmacology.* 2020 Feb; 28(1): 1–18.

Harikumar, K., et al. "Inhibition of viral carcinogenesis by *Phyllanthus amarus.*" *Integr. Cancer Ther.* 2009 Sep; 8(3): 254–60.

Harikumar, K., et al. "*Phyllanthus amarus* inhibits cell growth and induces apoptosis in Dalton's lymphoma ascites cells through activation of caspase-3 and downregulation of Bcl-2." *Integr. Cancer Ther.* 2009 Jun; 8(2): 190–4.

Huang, S., et al. "Anti-cancer effects of *Phyllanthus urinaria* and relevant mechanisms." *Chang. Gung. Med. J.* 2010 Sep–Oct; 33(5): 477–87.

Huang, S., et al. "Ellagic acid, the active compound of *Phyllanthus urinaria,* exerts *in vivo* anti-angiogenic effect and inhibits MMP-2 activity." *Evid. Based. Complement. Alternat. Med.* 2011; 2011: 215035.

Huang, S., et al. "*Phyllanthus urinaria* increases apoptosis and reduces telomerase activity in human nasopharyngeal carcinoma cells." *Forsch. Komplementmed.* 2009 Feb; 16(1): 34–40.

Jia, L., et al. "A potential anti-tumor herbal medicine, Corilagin, inhibits ovarian cancer cell growth through blocking the TGF-β signaling pathways." *BMC Complement. Altern. Med.* 2013 Feb; 13: 33.

Jia, L., et al. "Corilagin sensitizes epithelial ovarian cancer to chemotherapy by inhibiting Snail Oglycolysis pathways." *Oncol. Rep.* 2017 Oct; 38(4): 2464–2470.

Ko, H. "Geraniin inhibits TGF-β1-induced epithelial-mesenchymal transition and suppresses A549 lung cancer migration, invasion and anoikis resistance." *Bioorg. Med. Chem. Lett.* 2015 Sep; 25(17): 3529–34.

Lee, S., et al. "Antimetastatic effects of *Phyllanthus* on human lung (A549) and breast (MCF-7) cancer cell lines." *PLoS One.* 2011; 6(6): e20994.

Lee, S., et al. "Suppression of ERK1/2 and hypoxia pathways by four *Phyllanthus* species inhibits metastasis of human breast cancer cells." *J. Food Drug Anal.* 2016 Oct; 24(4): 855–865.

Leite, D., et al. "The cytotoxic effect and the multidrug resistance reversing action of lignans from *Phyllanthus amarus.*" *Planta Med.* 2006 Dec; 72(15): 1353–8.

Lim, W., et al. "Dioscin suppresses TGF-β1-induced epithelial-mesenchymal transition and suppresses A549 lung cancer migration and invasion." *Bioorg. Med. Chem. Lett.* 2017 Aug; 27(15): 3342–3348.

Lu, K., et al. "*Phyllanthus urinaria* suppresses human osteosarcoma cell invasion and migration by transcriptionally inhibiting u-PA via ERK and Akt signaling pathways." *Food Chem. Toxicol.* 2013 Feb; 52: 193–9.

Luan, B., et al. "Corilagin could help to overcome PARP inhibitor resistance by inhibiting ERK signaling pathways." *Cancer Res.* 2019 Jul; 70(13 Suppl): 3816.

Mellinger, C., et al. "Chemical and biological properties of an arabinogalactan from *Phyllanthus niruri.*" *J. Nat. Prod.* 2005; 68(10): 1479–83.

Mohamed, S. et al. "Dendritic cells pulsed with generated tumor cell lysate from *Phyllanthus amarus* Schum. & Thonn. induces anti-tumor immune response." *BMC Complement. Altern. Med.* 2018 Aug; 18(1): 232.

Navarro, M., et al. "Proanthocyanidin characterization, antioxidant and cytotoxic activities of three plants commonly used in traditional medicine in Costa Rica: *Petiveria alliaceae* L., *Phyllanthus niruri* L. and *Senna reticulata* Willd." *Plants.* 2017 Oct 19; 6(4).

Ng, K., et al. "Anti-angiogenic and cytotoxicity studies of some medicinal plants." *Planta Med.* 2010 Jun; 76(9): 935–40.

References

Nguyen, V., et al. "Cytotoxic activity of extracts and fractions from *Paramignya trimera* root and *Phyllanthus amarus* against pancreatic cancer cell lines." *J. Cancer Res. Ther.* 2019 Jan–Mar; 15(1): 245–249.

Nguyen, V., et al. "Physicochemical properties, antioxidant and cytotoxic activities of crude extracts and fractions from *Phyllanthus amarus.*" *Medicines.* 2017 Jun 18; 4(2).

Ooi, K., et al. "Cytotoxic, caspase-3 induction and *in vivo* hepatoprotective effects of phyllanthin, a major constituent of *Phyllanthus niruri,*" *J. Funct. Foods.* 2015; 14: 236–243.

Paul, S., et al. "Lignan enriched fraction (LRF) of *Phyllanthus amarus* promotes apoptotic cell death in human cervical cancer cells *in vitro.*" *Sci. Rep.* 2019 Oct; 9(1): 14950.

Prajapati, A., et al. "Effect of *Phyllanthus amarus* on serum biochemical changes in azaserine induced pancreatic cancer in Wistar rats." *Vet. World.* 2015 Aug; 8(8): 937–40.

Priyal, S., and Satheeshkumar, P. "Chapter 5. Natural products from plants: Recent developments in phytochemicals, phytopharmaceuticals, and plant-based nutraceuticals as anticancer agents." in *Functional and Preservative Properties of Phytochemicals.* 2020 Academic Press. pages 145–163.

Puspital, N., et al. "The effect of *Phyllanthus niruri* L extracts on human leukemic cell proliferation and apoptosis induction." *Indones. J. Pharm.* 2019 Nov; 30(4): 241.

Qui, F., et al. "Corilagin inhibits esophageal squamous cell carcinoma by inducing DNA damage and down-regulation of RNF8." *Anticancer Agents Med. Chem.* 2019; 19(8): 1021–1028.

Rajeshkumar, N. "Antitumour and anticarcinogenic activity of *Phyllanthus amarus* extract." *J. Ethnopharmacol.* 2002; 81(1): 17–22.

Raphael, K., et al. "Inhibition of N-Methyl N′-nitro-N-nitrosoguanidine (MNNG) induced gastric carcinogenesis by *Phyllanthus amarus* extract." *Asian Pac. J. Cancer Prev.* 2006 Apr–Jun; 7(2): 299–302.

Sawitri, E. "Apoptosis of colorectal cancer cell on Sprague-Dawley rats induced with 1, 2 dimethylhidrazine and *Phyllanthus niruri* Linn extract." *Int. J. Sci. Eng.* 2016; 10: 45–50.

Sharma, P., et al. "Anti-tumor activity of *Phyllanthus niruri* (a medicinal plant) on chemical-induced skin carcinogenesis in mice." *Asian Pac. J. Can. Prevent.* 2009; 10: 1089–1094.

Sharma, P., et al. "Modulatory influence of *Phyllanthus niruri on* oxidative stress, antioxidant defense and chemically induced skin tumors." *J. Environ. Pathol. Toxicol. Oncol.* 2011; 30(1): 43–53.

Silva, M., et al. "UPLC-HRMS and NMR applied in the evaluation of solid-phase extraction methods as a rational strategy of dereplication of *Phyllanthus spp.* aiming at the discovery of cytotoxic metabolites." *J. Chromatogr. B. Analyt. Technol. Biomed. Life Sci.* 2019 Jul; 1120: 51–61.

Sparzak, B., et al. "Cytotoxic lignan from the non-transformed root culture of *Phyllanthus amarus*." *Molecules*. 2015 Apr; 20(5): 7915–24.

Sripanidkulchai, B., et al. "Antimutagenic and anticarcinogenic effects of *Phyllanthus amarus*." *Phytomedicine*. 2002; 9(1): 26–32.

Tang, Y. et al. "*Phyllanthus spp.* exerts anti-angiogenic and anti-metastatic effects through inhibition on matrix metalloproteinase enzymes." *Nutr. Cancer*. 2015; 67(5): 783–95.

Tang, Y., et al. "Inhibition of MAPKs, Myc/Max, NFκB, and hypoxia pathways by *Phyllanthus* prevents proliferation, metastasis and angiogenesis in human melanoma (MeWo) cancer cell line." *Int. J. Med. Sci.* 2014 Apr; 11(6): 564–77.

Tang, Y., et al. "*Phyllanthus spp.* induces selective growth inhibition of PC-3 and MeWo human cancer cells through modulation of cell cycle and induction of apoptosis." *PLoS One*. 2010 Sep 8; 5(9): e12644.

Tang, Y., et al. "*Phyllanthus* suppresses prostate cancer cell, PC-3, proliferation and induces apoptosis through multiple signalling pathways (MAPKs, PI3K/Akt, NFκB, and Hypoxia)." *Evid. Based Complement. Alternat. Med.* 2013; 2013: 609581.

Tseng, H., et al. "Antimetastatic potentials of *Phyllanthus urinaria* L on A549 and Lewis lung carcinoma cells via repression of matrix-degrading proteases." *Integr. Cancer Ther.* 2012 Sep; 11(3): 267–78.

Wu, H., et al. "*Phyllanthus urinaria* induces apoptosis in human osteosarcoma 143B cells via activation of Fas/FasL- and mitochondria-mediated pathways." *Evid. Based Complement. Alternat. Med.* 2012; 2012: 925824.

Zheng, Z., et al. "Bioguided fraction and isolation of the antitumor components from *Phyllanthus niruri* L." *Biomed. Res. Int.* 2016: 9729275.

Diuretic Actions

Devi, M., et al. "Effect of *Phyllanthus niruri* on the diuretic activity of Punarnava tablets." *J. Res. Educ. Indian Med.* 1986; 5(1): 11–13.

Hnatyszyn, O., et al. "Diuretic activity of an aqueous extract of *Phyllanthus sellowianus*." *Phytomedicine*. 1999 Jul; 6(3): 177–179.

Saravanan, M., et al. "*In-vitro* qualitative and quantitative analysis of certain nutraceuticals as diuretic and antioxidant for hepatobiliary disorders (HBD)." *Int. J. Pharma Sci. Res.* 2014 Dec; 5(2): 896–902.

Srividya, N., et al. "Diuretic, hypotensive and hypoglycaemic effect of *Phyllanthus amarus*." *Indian J. Exp. Bio.* 1995 Oct; 33(11): 861–864.

Udupa, A., et al. "Diuretic activity of *Phyllanthus niruri* (Linn.) in rats." *Health* 2010; 2: 511–512.

Ueno, H., et al. "Chemical and pharmaceutical studies on medicinal plants in Paraguay, geraniin, an angiotensin-converting enzyme inhibitor from "parapa-rai mi" *Phyllanthus niruri.*" *J. Nat. Prod.* 1988; 51(2): 357–359.

Unander, D., et al. "Usage and bioassays in *Phyllanthus* (Euphorbiaceae). IV. Clustering of antiviral uses and other effects." *J. Ethnopharmacol.* 1995; 45: 1–18.

Yao, A., et al. "The acute diuretic effect of an ethanolic fraction of *Phyllanthus amarus* (Euphorbiaceae) in rats involves prostaglandins." *BMC Complement. Altern. Med.* 2018; 18: 94.

Yao, N., et al. "Comparative effects of aqueous extract of *Phyllanthus amarus* and its fractions on urinary excretion in rat." *J. Phytopharmacol.* 2016; 5: 182–184.

Hair Growth Actions

Gupta, R., et al. "Pharmacological investigation of hair growth promotional potential of *Phyllanthus niruri* Linn. extract against doxorubicin induced alopecia in experimental rats." *Int. J. Pharm. Life Sci.* 2018 Dec; 9(11/12): 5977–5984.

Luliana, S., et al. "Test activity of hair tonic of ethyl acetate fraction from the ethanol extract of meniran (*Phyllanthus niruri* L.) as hair grower to male white rat *(Rattus norvegicus)* wistar strain." *Res. J. Pharm. Tech.* 2019; 12(3): 999–1002.

Luliana, S., et al. "The influence of menthol in ethanol extract of meniran gel (*Phyllanthus niruri* L.) as a hair growth promoter in male Wistar rats." *Trad. Med. J.* 2019 Jan-Apr; 24(1): 1–8.

Nahata, A., et al. "Evaluation of 5a-reductase inhibitory activity of certain herbs useful as antiandrogens." *Andrologia.* 2014 Aug; 46(6): 592–601.

Patel, S., et al. "Evaluation of hair growth promoting activity of *Phyllanthus niruri.*" *Avicenna J. Phytomed.* 2015 Nov–Dec; 5(6): 512–9.

Wound Healing Actions

Devi, V., et al. "Effect of *Phyllanthus niruri* on wound healing in rats." *Indian J. Physiol Pharmacol.* 2005 Oct-Dec; 49(4): 487–90.

Shanbhag, T., et al. "Effect of *Phyllanthus niruri* Linn on burn wound in rats." *Asian Pac. J. Trop. Med.* 2010 Nov; 105–108.

Venkateshwarlu, G., et al. "Wound healing activity of *Phyllanthus niruri* in albino Wistar rats." *Asian J. of Chem.* 2012; 24(9): 3929–3930.

Chapter 5. A Consumer Guide for Chanca Piedra

Khatoon, S., et al. "Comparative pharmacognostic studies of three *Phyllanthus* species." *J. Ethnopharmacol.* 2006 Mar; 104(1-2): 79–86.

Kosnayani, A., "A qualitative analysis of tannin type and tannin content in meniran tea (*Phyllanthus niruri* Linn.) with permanganometry method." *Adv. Health Sci. Res.* 2019 Nov; 13: 15–19.

Safety and Toxicity Studies

Asare, G., et al. "Male rat hormone imbalance, testicular changes and toxicity associated with aqueous leaf extract of an antimalarial plant: *Phyllanthus niruri.*" *Pharm. Biol.* 2013 Jun; 51(6): 691–9.

Asare, G. et al. "Genotoxicity, cytotoxicity and toxicological evaluation of whole plant extracts of the medicinal plant *Phyllanthus niruri* (Phyllanthaceae)." *Genet. Mol. Res.* 2012 Jan; 11(1): 100–11.

Asare, G. et al. "Acute toxicity studies of aqueous leaf extract of *Phyllanthus niruri.*" *Interdiscip. Toxicol.* 2011 Dec; 4(4): 206–10.

Bakare, A., et al. "*In vivo* evaluation of genetic and systemic toxicity of aqueous extracts of *Phyllanthus amarus* in mice and rats." *Int. J. Toxicol. Pharmacol, Res.* 2015; 7(4): 1–9.

Darmawan, E., et al. "The sub-chronic toxicity test of meniran (*Phyllanthus niruri* L.) and pegagan (*Centella asiatica*) extract in Wistar strain rats on liver and kidney function." *J. Pharm. Sci. Com.* 2019 Nov; 16(2): 86–95.

Legba, B., et al. "Toxicological characterization of six plants of the Beninese Pharmacopoeia used in the treatment of Salmonellosis." *J. Toxicol.* 2019 Jul; 2019: 3530659.

Tangpukdee, N., et al. "Phase-I clinical trial to evaluate the safety and tolerability of oral SN-1 extract formulation in healthy Thai volunteers." *J. Trop. Med. Parasitol.* 2004; 27: 71–78.

Possible Herb-Drug Interactions

Kumar, K., et al. "Inhibition of drug metabolizing enzymes (cytochrome P450) *in vitro* as well as *in vivo* by *Phyllanthus amarus* Schum & Thonn." *Biol. Pharm. Bull.* 2006; 29(7): 1310–3. Taesotikul, T., et al. "Effects of *Phyllanthus amarus* on the pharmacokinetics of midazolam and cytochrome P450 activities in rats." *Xenobiotica.* 2012 Jul; 42(7): 641–8.

Taesotikul, T., et al. "Inhibitory effects of *Phyllanthus amarus* and its major lignans on human microsomal cytochrome P450 activities: evidence for CYP3A4 mechanism-based inhibition." *Drug Metab. Pharmacokinet.* 2011; 26(2): 154–61.

About the Author

Leslie Taylor is one of the world's leading experts on rainforest medicinal plants. She founded, managed, and directed the Raintree group of companies from 1995 to 2012, and was a leader in creating a worldwide market for the important medicinal plants of the Amazon rainforest.

Having survived a rare form of leukemia only because of alternative health and herbal medicine, Leslie has been researching, studying, and documenting alternative healing modalities—including herbal medicine—for more than thirty years. A dedicated herbalist and naturopath, she developed many herbal formulas and remedies for her companies, for practitioners, and for individuals needing help. In 1995, while researching alternative AIDS and cancer therapies in Europe, Leslie became aware of a medicinal plant from the Peruvian rainforest called cat's claw. This research took her to the Peruvian rainforest to gain firsthand knowledge about this new medicinal plant. Upon her return, she founded Raintree Nutrition, Inc., to make this important rainforest medicinal plant and others available in the United States.

After that first trip, Leslie returned to the Amazon numerous times, continuing to research and document more rainforest medicinal plants. In these endeavors, she worked directly with indigenous Indian shamans and healers, learning about their use of healing plants, as well as with indigenous tribal communities and other rainforest communities. She also worked with phytochemists, botanists, ethnobotanists, researchers, and alternative and integrative health practitioners to document, research, test, and validate rainforest medicinal plants.

In 2012, with many other companies selling the rainforest plants that she had introduced to the United States, she decided to close her business and naturopathic practice and devote herself to educating people about the benefits of medicinal plants. She freely shared all her proprietary formulas by posting them on the Raintree website so that anyone can make and use them.

Now, Leslie Taylor remains a trusted source of factual information about rainforest medicinal plants and continues to update the Tropical Plant Database for these purposes. A practicing board certified naturopath for many years (now retired), she has lectured and taught classes in naturopathic medicine, herbal medicine, and ethnobotany, as well as environmental and sustainability issues in the Amazon rainforest. She is the author of *Herbal Secrets of the Rainforest* and of the best-selling *The Healing Power of Rainforest Herbs*, as well as the highly popular and extensively referenced Raintree Tropical Plant Database (http://www.rain-tree.com/plants.htm), which has been online since 1996. More information about Leslie Taylor and her other books can be found at http://rain-tree.com/author.htm and on her Amazon Author Page. She also has a personal blog where you can ask questions and share your results using chanca piedra with others at http://leslie-taylor-raintree.blogspot.com.

Made in the USA
San Bernardino, CA
21 April 2020